The Cambridge Dictionary of
Statistics in the Medical Sciences

The Cambridge Dictionary of Statistics in the Medical Sciences

B. S. EVERITT

CAMBRIDGE
UNIVERSITY PRESS

Published by the Press Syndicate of the University of Cambridge
The Pitt Building, Trumpington Street, Cambridge CB2 1RP
40 West 20th Street, New York, NY 10011-4211, USA
10 Stamford Road, Oakleigh, Melbourne 3166, Australia

First published 1995

Printed in Great Britain by Biddles Ltd, Guildford & King's Lynn.

A catalogue record for this book is available from the British Library

Library of Congress cataloguing in publication data

Everitt, Brian.
A dictionary of statistics in the medical sciences / B. S. Everitt.
p. cm.
ISBN 0-521-47382-9 (hc). – ISBN 0-521-47928-2 (pb)
1. Medical statistics–Dictionaries. I. Title.
RA407.E94 1996
610′.21–dc20 95–16562 CIP

ISBN 0 521 47382 9 hardback
ISBN 0 521 47928 2 paperback

To Joanna and Rachel

KW

Some thoughts on compilers of dictionaries (all from Samuel Johnson)
Lexicographer: a writer of dictionaries, a harmless drudge.

To make dictionaries is dull work.

But these were the dreams of a poet doomed at last to wake a lexicographer.

Sources

Of the many books examined in the process of compiling this dictionary, particular mention needs to be made of the following works that were extremely valuable for checking the definitions of many terms:

- *A Dictionary of Epidemiology* (Oxford University Press, 1988)
- *Dictionary of Basic Statistics* (Dover Publications, 1965)
- *A Dictionary of Statistical Terms* (Longman Scientific and Technical, 1990)
- *Encyclopedia of Statistical Science* (John Wiley and Sons, 1982)

Preface

During the last twenty years statistical methods have become of central importance in research studies in medicine and related disciplines, and also in day-to-day clinical practice. The medical literature is now liberally punctuated not only with relatively routine statistical terms such as *P-values*, *t-tests*, *confidence intervals*, and *linear regression*, but also with the more exotic and esoteric language of the discipline, for example, *hazard function*, *empirical Bayes method* and *autoregressive moving-average models*. In addition, specialist medical statistics journals are now available that contain accounts of important new methods, for example, *generalized estimating equations* and *artificial neural networks*, which, no doubt, will soon find their way into the general medical literature. In the hope that relatively brief explanations of the phrases in the expanding vocabulary of medical statistics will be welcomed by many, this dictionary provides definitions of approximately 2000 terms; these are primarily statistical but a number of relevant mathematical, computing and genetic terms are also included. Since other dictionaries of statistics not specific to medical science exist, definitions of *general* statistical terms given in this dictionary are, on the whole, shorter than those relating to statistical topics most relevant to medicine and associated disciplines. Many of the definitions contain some mathematical formulae and/or nomenclature. This is almost inevitable, but it is hoped that the accompanying written and, in some cases, graphical material, will still enable the less mathematically sophisticated reader to understand most of the concepts being described. Hopefully, this will mean that the material is useful not only to medical statisticians and students on applied statistics courses, but also to general medical researchers, health professionals and even clinicians.

Apart from complaints that terms are incorrectly or poorly defined, compilers of dictionaries are also open to criticism for their choice of which terms to include and which to exclude. Critics are often no more inclined to be sympathetic to the problems of arranging terms and cross-referencing. Convention requires that the lexicographer, partially at least, pre-empts such critics by asking for their help in correcting his or her mistakes by reporting omissions, etc., so that they can be included in future editions of the work. (Lexicographers may be dull but they need to be optimistic!) Not all settle for this convention, however, and I am tempted to take the advice of another dictionary writer, Professor Stuart

Sutherland, for dealing with such criticism. In the preface of his excellent *Dictionary of Psychology* (although I have doubts about his definition of *love*!), Professor Sutherland makes the following plea:

> *It is customary for dictionary writers to acknowledge that their work is likely to contain mistakes, and to ask readers to write pointing out any they encounter. I apologise for any errors that have crept into mine, but I beg the reader not to draw my attention to them. It was depressing enough searching out the technical vocabulary in psychology and related subjects without having to learn at the end of it all that I got everything wrong.*

But being a statistician, a profession whose members are, on the whole, more conventional than their counterparts from psychology, I would appeal to those readers who identify an obvious exclusion, or a poor definition, to let me have the details. And being not only conventional but also optimistic, I can promise them a mention in future editions.

B. S. Everitt, Institute of Psychiatry

Notes on use

Several forms of cross-referencing are used. Terms in *slanted roman* in an entry appear as a separate headword, although headwords defining very commonly occurring terms such as **variable**, **population**, **sample**, **mean**, **normality**, **significance level**, **degrees of freedom**, **mortality**, **explanatory variable**, etc., are *not* referred to in this way. Some entries simply refer readers to another entry. This may indicate that the terms are synonyms, or, alternatively, that the term is more conveniently discussed under another entry. In the latter case the term is printed in *italics* in the main entry.

Entries are in alphabetical order using the letter-by-letter rather than the word-by-word convention. In terms containing numbers or Greek letters, the numbers or corresponding English word are spelt out and alphabetized accordingly. So, for example, 2×2 table is found under **two-by-two table**, and α- trimmed mean, under **alpha-trimmed mean**. No headings are inverted, for example, there is an entry under **Box–Müller transformation** *not* under **Transformation, Box-Müller**.

Acknowledgements

Several people were kind enough to supply definitions of particular terms and/or to suggest terms that should be included. I am grateful in this respect to Edward Bullmore (particular thanks are due to 'Ed'), Geoff Der, Graham Dunn, David Hand, Andrew Pickles and Pak Sham. Many more people, the authors of the large number of papers, articles and books examined while compiling this dictionary, unwittingly provided the basis of many of the definitions included. To these unnamed souls, many thanks. I am also indebted to David Tranah of Cambridge University Press for several suggestions which considerably improved the dictionary, and for his support and encouragement during its preparation. In addition the reports of two anonymous referees were very helpful.

Lastly, for showing tolerance beyond the call of duty when asked to share the author's enthusiasm for the discovery of *quangle*, *Pickles plot*, etc., Mary Elizabeth Bennett receives my upmost gratitude.

A

Aalen plot: A diagnostic tool for the assessment of time-dependent effects amongst the covariates in a *Cox's proportional hazards model.*

Ability parameter: See **Rasch model**.

Abortion rate: The annual number of abortions per 1000 women of reproductive age (usually defined as age 15–44 years).

Absolute deviation: Synonym for **average deviation.**

Absolute risk: Synonym for **incidence**.

Absorbing barrier: See **random walk**.

Accelerated failure time model: A general model for data consisting of *survival times*, in which explanatory variables measured on an individual are assumed to act multiplicatively on the time-scale, and so affect the rate at which an individual proceeds along the time axis. Consequently, the model can be interpreted in terms of the speed of progression of a disease. In the simplest case of comparing two groups of patients, for example, on different treatments, this model assumes that the survival time of an individual on one treatment is a multiple of the survival time on the other treatment; as a result the probability that an individual on treatment one survives beyond time t is the probability that an individual on treatment two survives beyond time ϕt, where ϕ is an unknown positive constant. When the endpoint of interest is the death of a patient, values of ϕ less than unity correspond to an acceleration in the time of death of an individual assigned to treatment one, and values of ϕ greater than unity indicate the reverse. The parameter ϕ is known as the *acceleration factor*.

Acceleration factor: See **accelerated failure time model**.

Acceptable quality level: See **quality control procedures.**

Acceptable risk: The risk for which the benefits of a particular medical procedure are considered to outweigh the potential hazards.

Acceptance region: The set of values of a *test statistic* for which the *null hypothesis* is accepted.

Acceptance sampling: A type of *quality control procedure* in which a sample is taken from a collection or batch of items, and the decision to accept the batch as satisfactory, or reject it as unsatisfactory, is based on the proportion of defective items in the sample.

Accidently empty cells: Synonym for **sampling zeros**.

Accuracy: The degree of conformity to some recognized standard value. See also **bias**.

ACE: Abbreviation for **alternating conditional expectation**.

ACF: Abbreviation for **autocorrelation function**.

Action lines: See **quality control procedures**.

Active control equivalence studies: Studies directed toward demonstrating that an experimental treatment is equivalent in efficacy to a standard therapy. The justification for running such trials is that even if the new treatment is no better than the existing standard, it may still be useful for patients who are resistant to, or who simply cannot tolerate, the standard treatment.

Active control trials: *Clinical trials* in which the trial drug is compared with some other active compound rather than a placebo.

Activities of daily living scale (ADLS): A scale designed to measure physical ability/disability that is used in investigations of various chronic disabling conditions such as arthritis. The scale is based on scores for responses to questions about mobility, self-care, grooming, etc. See also **Barthel index** and **health assessment questionnaire**.

Actuarial statistics: The statistics used by actuaries to evaluate risks, calculate liabilities and plan the financial course of insurance, pensions, etc. An example is *life expectancy* for people of various ages, occupations, etc. See also **life table**.

Adaptation: A heritable component of the *phenotype* which confers an advantage in survival and reproductive success. The process by which organisms adapt to environmental conditions.

Adaptive cluster sampling: A procedure in which an initial set of subjects is selected by some sampling procedure and, whenever the variable of interest of a selected subject satifies a given criterion, additional subjects in the neighbourhood of that subject are added to the sample.

Adaptive design: A rarely used design for *clinical trials* in which the treatment a patient receives depends to some extent on the response to treatment of previous patients in the trial. The aim is to diminish the proportion of patients being given the 'inferior' treatment as the trial proceeds.

Adaptive methods: Procedures that use various aspects of the sample data to select the most appropriate type of statistical method for analysis. For example, the sample *skewness* might be calculated and, depending on its value, either the mean or the median of the sample used as a measure of location.

Adaptive sampling: A sampling procedure in which the selection process depends on the observed values of some variable of interest. The main aim of such schemes is to achieve gains in precision or efficiency compared with conventional designs.

Added variable plot: A graphical procedure used in all types of *regression analysis* for identifying whether or not a particular explanatory variable should be included in a model, in the presence of other explanatory variables. The variable that is the candidate for inclusion in the model may be new, or it may simply be a higher power of one currently included. If the candidate variable is denoted x_i, then the *residuals* from the regression of the response variable on all the explanatory variables, save x_i, are plotted against the residuals from the regression of x_i on the remaining explanatory variables. A strong linear relationship in the plot indicates the need for x_i in the regression equation. (See Fig. 1 opposite.)

Addition rule for probabilities: For two events, A and B, that are *mutually exclusive*, the probability of either event occurring is the sum of the individual probabilities, i.e.,

$$P(A \text{ or } B) = P(A) + P(B)$$

where $P(A)$ denotes the probability of event A etc. For k mutually exclusive events, $A_1, A_2, \ldots, A_k$, the more general rule is

$$P(A_1 \text{ or } A_2 \text{ or } \ldots A_k) = P(A_1) + P(A_2) + \ldots + P(A_k).$$

Additive effect: A term used when the effect of administering two treatments together is the sum of their separate effects. See also **additive model**.

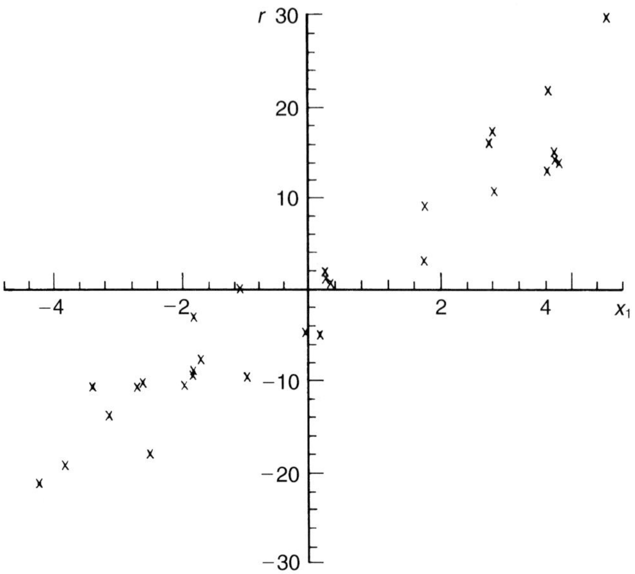

Fig 1 Added variable plot indicating a variable that should be included in the model.

Additive genetic variance: The variance of a characteristic that can be explained by the additive effects of genes.

Additive model: A model in which the explanatory variables have an *additive effect* on the response variable. So, for example, if variable A has an effect of size a on some response measure and variable B one of size b on the same response, then in an assumed additive model for A and B their combined effect would be $a + b$.

Adequate subset: A term used in *regression analysis* for a subset of the explanatory variables that is thought to contain as much information about the response variable as the complete set. See also **selection methods in regression**.

Adherence: Synonym for **compliance**.

Adjacency matrix: A matrix with elements, x_{ij}, used to indicate the connections in a *directed graph*. If node i relates to node j, $x_{ij} = 1$, otherwise $x_{ij} = 0$.

Adjectival scales: Scales with adjectival descriptions and discrete or continous responses. Two examples are,

(a) Discrete response

How much pain are you suffering today?

below average average above average

(b) Continuous response

How satisfied were you with your treatment?

|———————|———————|———————|———————|———————|

very dissatisfied dissatisfied neutral satisfied very satisfied

See also **visual analogue scales**.

Adjusted treatment means: Estimates of the treatment means in an *analysis of covariance*, after adjusting all treatments to the same mean level for the covariate(s), using the estimated relationship between the covariate(s) and the response variable.

Adjusting for baseline: The process of allowing for the effect of *baseline characteristics* on the response variable, usually in the context of a *clinical trial*. A number of methods might be used, for example, the analysis of simple *change scores*, the analysis of percentage change, or, in some cases, the analysis of more complicated variables, such as 100 × change/baseline. In general, it is preferable to use the adjusted variable that has least dependence on the baseline measure. In the context of a *longitudinal study* in which the correlations between the repeated measures over time are moderate to large, then using the baseline values as covariates in an *analysis of covariance* is known to be more efficient than analysing change scores. See also **baseline balance**.

ADLS: Abbreviation for **activities of daily living scale**.

Adverse event: Any undesirable event experienced by a subject during a *clinical trial*, irrespective of the relationship to the study treatment.

Age-dependent birth–death process: A *birth–death process* where the *birth rates* and *death rates* are not constant over time, but change in a manner which is dependent on the age of the individual.

Age heaping: A term applied to the collection of data on ages when these are accurate only to the nearest year or half year.

Age-incidence curve: Plots of age against the *age-specific incidence rate* for some disease of interest.

Age–period–cohort model: A model important in many *observational studies* when it is reasonable to suppose that age, number of years exposed to *risk factor*, and age when first exposed to risk factor, all contribute to disease risk. Unfortunately all three factors cannot be entered simultaneously into a model since this would result in *collinearity*, because 'age first exposed to risk factor' + 'years exposed to risk factor' is equal to 'age'. Various methods have been suggested for disentangling the dependence of the factors, although most commonly one of the factors is simply not included in the modelling process.

Age–sex register: A list of of all members of a medical practice classified by age and sex.

Age-specific death rates: Death rates calculated within a number of relatively narrow age bands. For example, for 20–30 year olds,

$$\mathrm{DR}_{20,30} = \frac{\text{number of deaths among } 20-30 \text{ year olds in a year}}{\text{average population size in } 20-30 \text{ year olds in the year}}$$

Calculating death rates in this way is usually necessary since such rates almost invariably differ widely with age, a variation not reflected in the *crude death rate*. See also **cause-specific death rates**.

Age-specific failure rate: Synonym for **hazard function**.

Age-specific incidence rates: *Incidence rates* calculated within a number of relatively narrow age bands. See also **age-specific death rates**.

Agglomerative hierachical clustering methods: Methods of *cluster analysis* that begin with each individual in a separate cluster and then, in a series of steps, combine individuals and later, clusters, into new, larger clusters until a final stage is reached where all individuals are members of a single group. At each stage the individuals or clusters that are 'closest', according to some particular definition of distance are joined. The whole process can be summarized by a *dendrogram*. Solutions corresponding to particular numbers of clusters are found by 'cutting' the dendrogram at the appropriate level. See also **average linkage, complete linkage, single linkage, Ward's method, Mojena's test, K-means cluster analysis** and **divisive methods**.

AI: Abbreviation for **artificial intelligence**.

AID: Abbreviation for **automatic interaction detector**.

Akaike's information criterion: An index used in a number of areas as an aid for choosing between competing models. It is defined as

$$-2L_m + 2m$$

where L_m is the maximized *log-likelihood* and m is the number of parameters in the model. The index takes into account both the statistical goodness of fit and the number of parameters that have to be estimated to achieve this particular degree of fit, by imposing a penalty for increasing the number of parameters. Lower values of the index indicate the preferred model, that is, the one with the fewest parameters that still provides an adequate fit to the data. See also **parsimony principle** and **Schwarz's criterion**.

Algorithm: A well-defined set of rules which, when routinely applied, lead to a solution of a particular class of mathematical or computational problem.

Alias: See **confounding**.

Allele: One of two or more gene types that may occur at a given location in the genes of an individual.

Allocation rule: See **discriminant analysis**.

Allometric growth: Changes in the shape of an organism associated with different growth rates of its parts.

Allometry: The quantitative study of the relationship between the size and shape of organisms.

All subsets regression: A form of *regression analysis* in which all possible models are considered and the 'best' selected by comparing the values of some appropriate criterion, for example, *Mallow's C_k statistic*, calculated on each. If there are q explanatory variables, there are a total of $2^q - 1$ models to be examined. The *leaps-and-bounds algorithm* is generally used, so that only a small fraction of the possible models have to be considered. See also **selection methods in regression** and **leaps-and-bounds algorithm**.

Alpha(α): The probability of a *type I error*. See also **significance level**.

Alpha(α)-trimmed mean: A method of estimating the mean of a population that is less affected by the presence of *outliers* than the usual estimator, namely the sample average. Calculating the statistic involves dropping a proportion α (approximately) of the observations from both ends of the sample before calculating the mean of the remainder. If $x_{(1)}, x_{(2)}, \cdots, x_{(n)}$ represent the ordered sample values, then the measure is given by

$$\alpha_{\text{trimmed mean}} = \frac{1}{n-2k}\sum_{i=k+1}^{n-k} x_{(i)}$$

where k is the smallest integer greater than or equal to αn. (Note that the term α in this definition is not that defined in the entry **alpha**).

Alpha(α)-Winsorized mean: A method of estimating the mean of a population that is less affected by the presence of *outliers* than the usual estimator, namely the sample average. Essentially the k smallest and k largest observations, where k is the smallest integer greater than or equal to αn, are reduced in size to the next remaining observation and counted as though they had these values. Specifically given by

$$\alpha\text{Winsorized mean} = \frac{1}{n}\left[(k+1)(x_{(k+1)} + x_{(n-k)}) + \sum_{i=k+2}^{n-k-1} x_{(i)}\right]$$

where $x_{(1)}, x_{(2)}, \cdots, x_{(n)}$ are the ordered sample values. (Note that the term α in this definition is not that defined in the entry **alpha**).

Alshuler's estimator: An estimator of the *survival function*, given by

$$\prod_{j=1}^{k} \exp(-d_j/n_j)$$

where d_j is the number of deaths at time $t_{(j)}$, n_j the number of individuals alive just before $t_{(j)}$, and $t_{(1)} \leq t_{(2)}, \cdots \leq t_{(k)}$ are the ordered *survival times*. See also **product limit estimator**.

Alternating conditional expectation (ACE): A procedure for estimating optimal transformations for *regression analysis* and correlation. Given *random variables* x and y, the method finds the transformations $g(y)$ and $s(x)$ that maximize the correlation between the transformed variables. The technique allows for arbitrary, smooth transformations of both response and explanatory variables.

Alternative hypothesis (H_1): The hypothesis against which the *null hypothesis* is tested.

Amersham model: A model used for *dose–response curves* in immunoassay and given by

$$y = 100(2(1-\beta_1)\beta_2)/(\beta_3 + \beta_2 + \beta_4 + x + [(\beta_3 - \beta_2 + \beta_4 + x)^2 + 4\beta_3\beta_2]^{\frac{1}{2}}) + \beta_1$$

where y is percentage binding and x is the analyte concentration. Estimates of the four parameters, $\beta_1, \beta_2, \beta_3, \beta_4$, may be obtained in a variety of ways.

Amplitude: A term used in relation to *time series*, for the value of the series at its peak or trough taken from some mean value or trend line.

Analysis as-randomized: Synonym for **intention-to-treat analysis**.

Analysis of covariance (ANCOVA): An extension of the *analysis of variance* that allows for the possible effects of covariates on the response variable, in addition to the effects of the factor or treatment variables. The covariates are assumed to be unaffected by treatments and, in general, their relationship to the response is assumed to be linear. Inclusion of covariates decreases the *error mean square* and hence increases the sensitivity of the *F-tests* used in assessing treatment differences. See also **parallelism in ANCOVA** and **generalized linear models**.

Analysis of dispersion: Synonym for **multivariate analysis of variance**.

Analysis of variance (ANOVA): The separation of variance attributable to one cause from the variance attributable to others. By partitioning the total variance of a set of observations into parts due to particular factors, for example, sex, treatment group, and comparing variances by way of *F-tests*, differences between means can be assessed. The simplest analysis of this type involves a *one way design*, in which N subjects are allocated, usually at random, to the k different levels of a single factor. The total variation in the observations is then divided into a part due to differences between level means (the *between groups sum of squares*) and a part due to the differences between subjects in the same group (the *within groups sum of squares*, also known as the *residual sum of squares*). These terms are usually arranged as an *analysis of variance table*.

Source	**df**	**SS**	**MS**	**MSR**
Bet. grps	$k-1$	SSB	$\text{SSB}/(k-1)$	$\frac{\text{SSB}/(k-1)}{\text{SSW}/(N-k)}$
With. grps	$N-k$	SSW	$\text{SSW}/(N-k)$	
Total	$N-1$			

SS = sum of squares; MS = mean square; MSR = mean square ratio.

If the means of the populations represented by the factor levels are the same, then the *between groups mean square* and *within groups mean square* are both estimates of the same population variance. Whether this is so can be assessed by a suitable F-test on the mean square ratio. See also **analysis of covariance, parallel groups design** and **factorial designs**.

Analysis of variance table: See **analysis of variance**.

Ancillary statistic: A statistic that contains no information about some parameter of interest.

ANCOVA: Acronym for **analysis of covariance**.

Anderson–Darling test: A test that a given sample of observations arises from some specified theoretical *probability distribution*. For testing the normality of the data, for example, the *test statistic* is

$$A_n^2 = -\frac{1}{n}\left[\sum_{i=1}^{n}(2i-1)\{\log z_i + \log(1 - z_{n+1-i})\}\right] - n$$

where $x_{(1)} \leq x_{(2)} \leq \cdots \leq x_{(n)}$ are the ordered observations, s^2 is the sample variance, and

$$z_i = \Phi\left(\frac{x_{(i)} - \bar{x}}{s}\right),$$

where

$$\Phi(x) = \int_{-\infty}^{x} \frac{1}{\sqrt{2\pi}} e^{-\frac{1}{2}u^2} du.$$

The null hypothesis of normality is rejected for 'large' values of A_n^2. *Critical values* of the test statistic are available. See also **Shapiro–Wilk test**.

Andrews' plots: A graphical display of *multivariate data*, in which an observation, $\mathbf{x}' = [x_1, x_2, \cdots, x_q]$, is represented by a function of the form

$$f_{\mathbf{x}}(t) = x_1/\sqrt{2} + x_2 \sin(t) + x_3 \cos(t) + x_4 \sin(2t) + x_5 \cos(2t) + \cdots$$

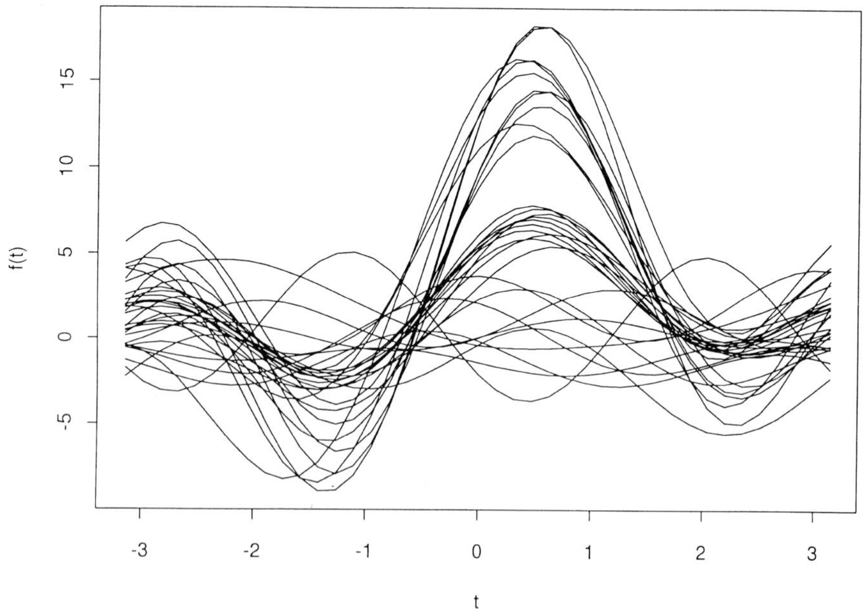

Fig 2 Andrews' plots for thirty, five-dimensional observations. Evidence for three 'clusters' shown by the three bands of plots at $t = 0.5$.

plotted over the range of values $-\pi \leq t \leq \pi$. A set of multivariate observations is displayed as a collection of these plots, and it can be shown that those functions that remain close together for all values of t correspond to observations that are close to one another in terms of their *Euclidean distance*. This property means that such plots can often be used to both detect groups of similar observations and identify *outliers* in multivariate data. The example shown consists of plots for a sample of 30 observations, each having five variable values. The plot indicates the presence of three groups in the data. See also **Chernoff's faces** and **glyphs**.

Angular transformation: Synonym for **arc sine transformation**.

Animal model: A study carried out in a population of laboratory animals that is used to model processes comparable to those that occur in human populations.

Annealing algorithm: A procedure that seeks the minimum of some deterministic objective function. The method operates by applying small perturbations to the current solution.

ANOVA: Acronym for **analysis of variance**.

Antagonism: See **synergism**.

Ante-dependence model: A model for *longitudinal data* which builds in *serial correlations* by allowing the error term for the jth repeated measure, e_j, to be dependent on a limited number of its predecessors, $e_{j-1}, \cdots, e_1$. The simplest such model would have e_j dependent only on e_{j-1}, and would essentially be equivalent to a *first order autoregressive model*.

Apgar score: See **Likert scales**.

A posteriori comparisons: Synonym for **post-hoc comparisons**.

Apparent error rate: Synonym for **resubstitution error rate**.

Approximation: A result that is not exact, but is sufficiently close for required purposes to be of practical use.

A priori comparisons: Synonym for **planned comparisons**.

Aranda–Ordaz transformations: A family of transformations for a proportion, p, given by

$$y = \ln\left[\frac{(1-p)^{-\alpha} - 1}{\alpha}\right]$$

When $\alpha = 1$, the formula reduces to the *logistic transformation* of p. As $\alpha \to 0$ the result is the *complementary log-log transformation*.

Arc sine transformation: A transformation for a proportion, p, designed to stabilize its variance, and produce values more suitable for techniques such as *analysis of variance* and *regression analysis*. The transformation is given by

$$y = \sin^{-1} \sqrt{p}$$

ARE: Abbreviation for **asymptotic relative efficiency**.

Area sampling: A method of sampling where a geographical region is subdivided into smaller areas (counties, villages, city blocks, etc.), some of which are selected at random, and the chosen areas are then subsampled or completely surveyed. See also **cluster sampling**.

Area under curve (AUC): Often a useful way of summarizing the information from a series of measurements made on an individual over time or for a *dose–response curve*. Usually calculated by adding the areas under the curve between each pair of consecutive observations, using, for example, the *trapezium rule*. See also $\mathbf{C}_{\max}$ and $\mathbf{T}_{\max}$.

ARIMA: Abbreviation for **autoregressive integrated moving-average model**.

Arithmetic mean: See **mean**.

ARMA: Abbreviation for **autoregressive moving-average model**.

Armitage–Doll model: A model of carcinogenesis in which the central idea is that the important variable determining the change in risk is not age, but time. The model proposes that cancer of a particular tissue develops according to the following process:

- a normal cell develops into a cancer cell by means of a small number of transitions through a series of intermediate steps;
- initially, the number of normal cells at risk is very large, and for each cell a transition is a rare event;
- the transitions are independent of one another.

Armitage–Hill test: A test for *carryover effect* in a *two-by-two crossover design* where the response is a *binary variable*.

Artificial intelligence (AI): A discipline that attempts to understand intelligent behaviour in the broadest sense, by getting computers to reproduce it, and to produce machines that behave intelligently, no matter what their underlying mechanism. (Intelligent behaviour is taken to include reasoning, thinking and learning.)

Artificial neural network: A mathematical structure modelled on the human neural network and designed to attack many statistical problems, particularly in the areas of *pattern recognition*, *multivariate analysis*, learning and memory. The essential feature of such a structure is a network of simple processing elements (*artificial neurons*) coupled together (either in the hardware or the software), so that they can cooperate. From a set of 'inputs' and an associated set of parameters the artificial neurons produce an 'output' that provides a possible solution to the problem under investigation. In many neural networks the relationship between the input received by a neuron and its output is determined by a *generalized linear model*.

Artificial neuron: See **artificial neural networks**.

Artificial pairing: See **paired samples**.

Ascertainment bias: A possible form of *bias*, particularly in *retrospective studies*, that arises from a relationship between the exposure to a *risk factor* and the probability of detecting an event of interest. In a study comparing women with cervical cancer and a control group, for example, an excess of oral contraceptive use amongst the cases might possibly be due to more frequent screening in this group.

ASN: Abbreviation for **average sample number**.

Assay: An experiment designed to estimate the strength, kind or quality of some physical, chemical, biological, physiological or psychological agent by means of the response induced by that agent in living or non-living matter. See also **bioassay**.

Assay run: A set of consecutive measurements, readings or observations all based on the same batch of reagents.

Assay validation: An assay method is considered validated if the accuracy (biasedness) and the precision (variability) of an assay result of a test sample (for example, amount of drug found, percentage of drug recovered or released) are within some acceptable limits. In particular for accuracy, with 95% assurance, the bias of an assay must be non-significant and has to be less than a certain percentage (for example, 5%) of the given standard at the worst case. For precision, the total variability, which includes the between run and within run variabilities, should give an estimated total *coefficient of variation* no greater than a specified percentage.

Assigned treatment: The treatment designated to be given to a patient in a *clinical trial*, as indicated at the time of enrolment.

Assignment method: Synonym for **discriminant analysis**.

Association: A general term used to describe the relationship between two variables. Essentially synonymous with correlation. Most often applied in the context of *binary variables* forming a *two-by-two contingency table*. See also **phi-coefficient** and **Goodman–Kruskal measures of association**.

Assumptions: The conditions under which statistical techniques give valid results. For example, *analysis of variance* generally assumes normality, homogeneity of variance and independence of the observations.

Asymmetrical distribution: A *probability distribution* or *frequency distribution* which is not symmetrical about some central value.

Asymmetric proximity matrices: *Proximity matrices* in which the off-diagonal elements, in the *i*th row and *j*th column and the *j*th row and *i*th column, are not necessarily equal. An example is provided by a matrix whose elements give the number of citations of one journal by another.

Asymptotically unbiased estimator: An *estimator* of a parameter which tends to being *unbiased* as the sample size (n) increases. For example,

$$s = \sqrt{\frac{1}{n-1}\sum_{i=1}^{n}(x_i - \bar{x})^2}$$

is not an unbiased estimator of the population standard deviation, but it is asymptotically unbiased.

Asymptotic distribution: The limiting *probability distribution* of a *random variable* calculated in some way from n other random variables, as $n \to \infty$. For example, the mean of n random variables from a *uniform distribution* has a *normal distribution* for large n.

Asymptotic method: Synonym for **large sample method**.

Asymptotic relative efficiency (ARE): The *relative efficiency* of two estimators of a parameter in the limit as the sample size increases.

Attachment level: A common measure of peridontal disease levels given by the minimum distance between the cement–enamel junction (a reference point on the tooth) and the epithelial attachment. Usually measured in millimetres with a graduated blunt-end probe.

Attack rate: A term often used for the *incidence* of a disease or condition in a particular group, or during a limited period of time, or under special circumstances such as an epidemic. A specific example would be one involving outbreaks of food poisoning, where the attack rates would be calculated for those people who have eaten a particular item and for those who have not.

Attenuation: A term applied to the correlation between two variables when both are subject to measurement error, to indicate that the value of the correlation between the 'true values' is likely to be underestimated. See also **regression dilution**.

Attributable risk: A measure of the association between exposure to a particular factor and the risk of a particular outcome, calculated as

$$\frac{\text{incidence rate among exposed} - \text{incidence rate among non-exposed}}{\text{incidence rate among exposed}}$$

Measures the amount of the *incidence* that can be attributed to one particular factor. See also **relative risk** and **prevented fraction**.

Attrition: A term used to describe the loss of subjects over the period of a *longitudinal study*. Such a phenomenon may cause problems in the analysis of data from such a study. See also **missing values**.

AUC: Abbreviation for **area under curve**.

Audit trail: A computer program that keeps a record of changes made to a **database**.

Autocorrelation: The internal correlation of the observations in a *time series*, usually expressed as a function of the time lag between observations. Also used for the correlations between points different distances apart in a set of *spatial data*. The autocorrelation at lag k, $\gamma(k)$, is defined mathematically as

$$\gamma(k) = \frac{E(X_t - \mu)(X_{t+k} - \mu)}{E(X_t - \mu)^2}$$

where $X_t, t = 0, \pm 1, \pm 2, \cdots$ represent the values of the series and μ is the mean of the series. E denotes *expected value*. The corresponding sample statistic is calculated as

$$\hat{\gamma}(k) = \frac{\sum_{t=1}^{n-k}(x_t - \bar{x})(x_{t+k} - \bar{x})}{\sum_{t=1}^{n}(x_t - \bar{x})^2}$$

where $\bar{x}$ is the mean of the series of observed values, $x_1, x_2, \cdots, x_n$. A plot of the sample values of the autocorrelation against the lag is known as the *autocorrelation function* or *correlogram* and is a basic tool in the

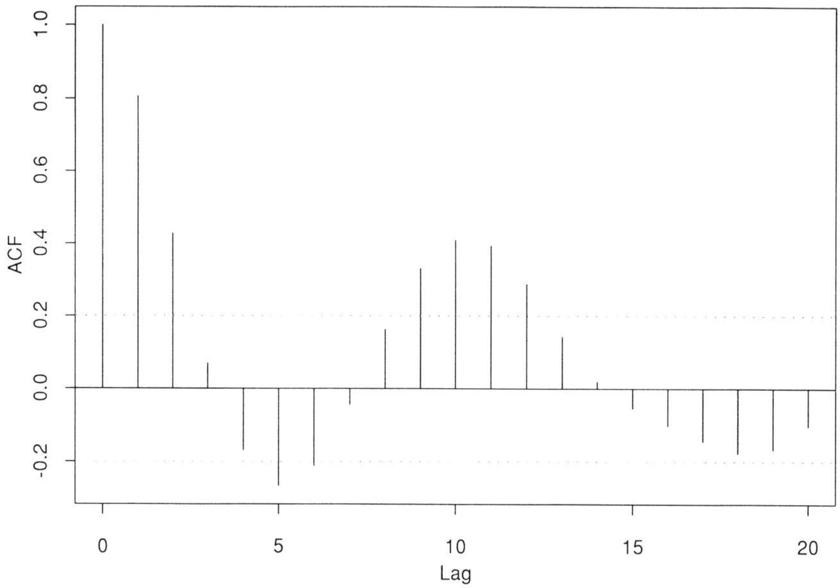

Fig 3 Correlogram plot.

analysis of time series, particularly for indicating possibly suitable models for the series. The term in the numerator of $\gamma(k)$ is the *autocovariance*. A plot of the autocovariance against lag is called the *autocovariance function*.

Autocorrelation function (ACF): See **autocorrelation**.

Autocovariance: See **autocorrelation**.

Autocovariance function: See **autocorrelation**.

Auto-encoding: Coding of clinical data by a computer program which matches original text to predetermined dictionary terms.

Automatic interaction detector (AID): A method that uses a set of categorical explanatory variables to divide data into groups that are relatively homogeneous with respect to the value of some response variable of interest. At each stage, the division of a group into two parts is defined by one of the explanatory variables, a subset of its categories defining one of the parts and the remaining categories the other part. Of the possible splits, the one chosen is that which maximizes the *between groups sum of squares* of the response variable. The groups eventually formed may often be useful in predicting the value of the response variable for some future observation. See also **classification and regression tree technique**.

Autoregressive integrated moving-average models (ARIMA): See **autoregressive moving-average model.**

Autoregressive model: A model used primarily in the analysis of *time series* in which the observation, x_t, at time t, is postulated to be a *linear function* of previous values of the series. So, for example, a *first order autoregressive model* is of the form

$$x_t = \phi x_{t-1} + a_t$$

where a_t is a random disturbance and ϕ is a parameter of the model. The corresponding model of order p is

$$x_t = \phi_1 x_{t-1} + \phi_2 x_{t-2} + \cdots + \phi_p x_{t-p} + a_t$$

which includes the p parameters, $\phi_1, \phi_2, \cdots, \phi_p$.

Autoregressive moving-average model (ARMA): A model for a *time series* that combines both an *autoregressive model* and a *moving-average model.* The general model of order p, q (usually denoted ARMA(p, q)) is

$$z_t = \phi_1 z_{t-1} + \phi_2 z_{t-2} + \cdots + \phi_p z_{t-p} + a_t - \theta_1 a_{t-1} - \cdots - \theta_q a_{t-q}$$

where $\phi_1, \phi_2, \cdots, \phi_p$ and $\theta_1, \theta_2, \cdots, \theta_q$ are the parameters of the model. In some cases such models are applied to the time series observations after *differencing* to achieve *a stationary series*, in which case they are known as *autoregressive integrated moving-average models.*

Available case analysis: An approach to handling *missing values* in a set of *multivariate data*, in which means, variances, covariances, etc., are calculated from all available subjects with non-missing values for the variable or pair of variables involved. Although this approach makes use of as much of the data as possible, it has disadvantages. One is that summary statistics will be based on different numbers of observations. More problematic, however, is that this method can lead to *variance–covariance matrices* and *correlation matrices* with properties that make them unsuitable for many methods of multivariate analysis such as *principal components analysis* and *factor analysis.*

Average: Most often used for the arithmetic mean of a sample of observations, but can also be used for other measures of location such as the median.

Average deviation: A little-used measure of the *spread* of a sample of observations. It is defined as

$$\text{Average deviation} = \frac{\sum_{i=1}^{n} |x_i - \bar{x}|}{n}$$

where $x_1, x_2, \cdots, x_n$ represent the sample values, and $\bar{x}$ their mean.

Average linkage: An *agglomerative hierarchical clustering method* that uses the average distance from members of one cluster to members of another cluster as the measure of inter-group distance.

Average sample number (ASN): A quantity used to describe the performance of a *sequential analysis*, given by the *expected value* of the sample size required to reach a decision to accept the *null hypothesis* or the *alternative hypothesis* and therefore to discontinue sampling.

B

Back projection: A term most often applied to a procedure for reconstructing plausible HIV *incidence* curves from AIDS incidence data. The method assumes that the *probability distribution* of the *incubation period* of AIDS has been estimated precisely from separate *cohort studies*, and uses this distribution to project the AIDS incidence data backwards to reconstruct an HIV *epidemic curve* that could plausibly have led to the observed AIDS incidence data.

Back-to-back stem-and-leaf plots: A method for comparing two distributions by 'hanging' the two sets of leaves in the *stem-and-leaf displays* of the two sets of data off the same stem. An example appears below.

Before									After		
				:	12	:	9				
				:	13	:	1	6			
		8	6	:	14	:	5	7	7		
			4	:	15	:	1	7			
9	7	2	0	:	16	:	5	6	8	8	
6	4	3	3	:	17	:	9				
		7	5	:	18	:	0				
			8	:	19	:					
			0	:	20	:	1				

Fig 4 Back-to-back stem-and-leaf plot for systolic blood pressure of fifteen subjects before and two hours after taking the drug captoril.

Backward elimination procedure: See **selection methods in regression**.

Backward-looking study: An alternative term for *retrospective study*.

Backward shift operator: A mathematical operator, denoted by B, met in the analysis of *time series*. When applied to a series, the operator moves the observations back one time unit, so that, if x_t represents the values of the series, then, for example,

$$Bx_t = x_{t-1}$$
$$B(Bx_t) = B(x_{t-1}) = x_{t-2}$$

Balaam's design: A design for testing differences between two treatments A and B in which patients are *randomly allocated* to one of four sequences, AA, AB, BA, or BB. See also **crossover design**.

Balanced design: A term usually applied to any *experimental design* in which the same number of observations is taken for each combination of the experimental factors.

Balanced incomplete block design: A design in which not all treatments are used in all *blocks*. Such designs have the following properties:

- Each block contains the same number of units,
- Each treatment occurs the same number of times in all blocks,
- Each pair of treatment combinations occurs together in a block the same number of times as any other pair of treatments.

In medicine, this type of design might be employed to avoid asking subjects to attend for treatment an unrealistic number of times, and thus possibly preventing problems with *missing values*. For example, in a study with five treatments (T_1, T_2, T_3, T_4, and T_5), it might be thought that subjects could realistically only be asked to make three visits. A possible balanced incomplete design in this case would be the following;:

Patient	**Visit 1**	**Visit 2**	**Visit 3**
1	T_4	T_5	T_1
2	T_4	T_2	T_5
3	T_2	T_4	T_1
4	T_5	T_3	T_1
5	T_3	T_4	T_5
6	T_2	T_3	T_1
7	T_3	T_1	T_4
8	T_3	T_5	T_2
9	T_2	T_3	T_4
10	T_5	T_1	T_2

Balanced longitudinal data: *Longitudinal data* for which observations at the same number of time points are available on each subject, and time intervals between pairs of corresponding observations are the same for all subjects. The observations need not be equally spaced.

Bar chart: A form of graphical representation for displaying data classified into a number of (usually unordered) categories. Equal-width rectangular bars are constructed over each category with height equal to the observed frequency of the category. See also **histogram** and **component bar chart**.

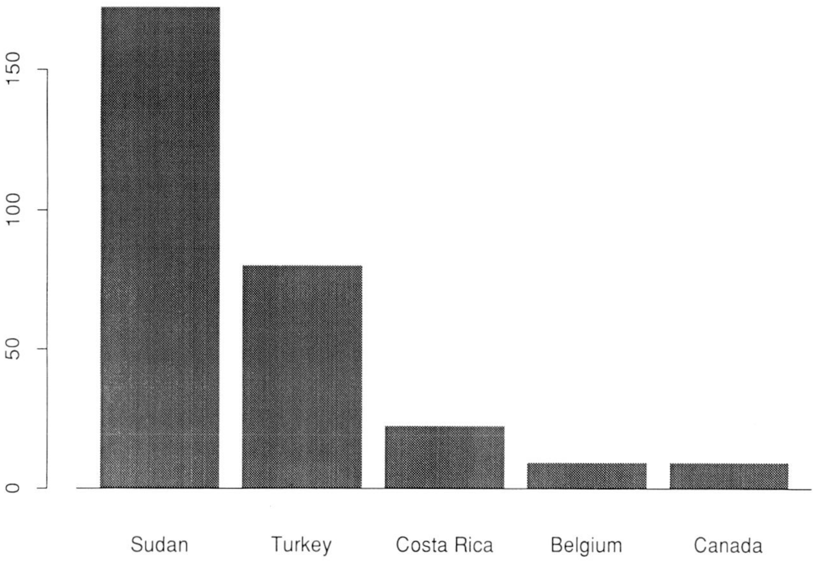

Fig 5 Bar chart of mortality rates per 1000 live births for children under five years of age in five different countries.

Barrett and Marshall model for conception: A biologically plausible model for the probability of conception in a particular menstrual cycle, which assumes that batches of sperm introduced on different days behave independently. The model is

$$P(\text{conception in cycle } k|\{X_{ik}\}) = 1 - \prod_i (1 - p_i)^{X_{ik}}$$

where the X_{ik} are 0,1 variables corresponding to whether there was intercourse or not on a particular day relative to the estimated day of ovulation (day 0). The parameter p_i is interpreted as the probability that conception would occur following intercourse on day i only. See also **EU model**.

Barthel index: A *quality-of-life variable* used to assess the ability of a patient to perform daily activities. A score of zero corresponds to complete dependence on others, a score of 100 implies that the patient can perform all usual daily activities without assistance. See also **activities of daily living scale**.

Bartlett's adjustment factor: A correction term for the *likelihood ratio* that makes the *chi-squared distribution* a more accurate approximation to its *probability distribution*.

Bartlett's test: A test for the equality of the variances of a number (k) of populations. The *test statistic* is given by

$$B = \left[\nu \ln s^2 + \sum_{i=1}^{k} \nu_i \ln s_i^2\right] / C$$

where s_i^2 is an estimate of the variance of population i based on ν_i degrees of freedom, and ν and s^2 are given by

$$\nu = \sum_{i=1}^{k} \nu_i$$

$$s^2 = \frac{\sum_{i=1}^{k} \nu_i s_i}{\nu}$$

and

$$C = 1 + \frac{1}{3(k-1)} \left[\sum_{i=1}^{k} \frac{1}{\nu_i} - \frac{1}{\nu}\right]$$

Under the hypothesis that the populations all have the same variance, B has a *chi-squared distribution* with $k - 1$ degrees of freedom. Sometimes used prior to applying *analysis of variance* techniques to assess the assumption of homogeneity of variance. Of limited practical value because of its known sensitivity to non-normality, so that a significant result might be due to departures from normality rather than to different variances. See also **Box's test** and **Hartley's test**.

Baseline balance: A term used to describe, in some sense, the equality of the observed *baseline characteristics* amongst the groups in, say, a *clinical trial*. Conventional practice dictates that, before proceeding to assess the treatment effects from the clinical outcomes, the groups must be shown to be comparable in terms of these baseline measurements and observations, usually by carrying out appropriate significant tests. Such tests are frequently criticized by statisticians who usually prefer important prognostic variables to be identified prior to the trial and then used in an *analysis of covariance*.

Baseline characteristics: Observations and measurements collected on subjects or patients at the time of entry into a study, before undergoing any treatment.

Baseline hazard function: See **Cox's proportional hazards model**.

BASIC: Acronym for Beginners All-purpose Symbolic Instruction Code, a programming language once widely used for writing microcomputer programs.

Basic reproduction rate: A term used in the theory of infectious diseases for the number of secondary cases which one case would produce in a completely susceptible population. The number depends on the duration of the *infectious period*, the probability of infecting a susceptible individual during one contact, and the number of new susceptible individuals contacted per unit time, with the consequence that it may vary considerably for different infectious diseases and also for the same disease in different populations.

Bathtub curve: The shape taken by the *hazard function* for the event of death in human beings; it is relatively high during the first year of life, decreases fairly soon to a minimum, and begins to climb again sometime around 45–50.

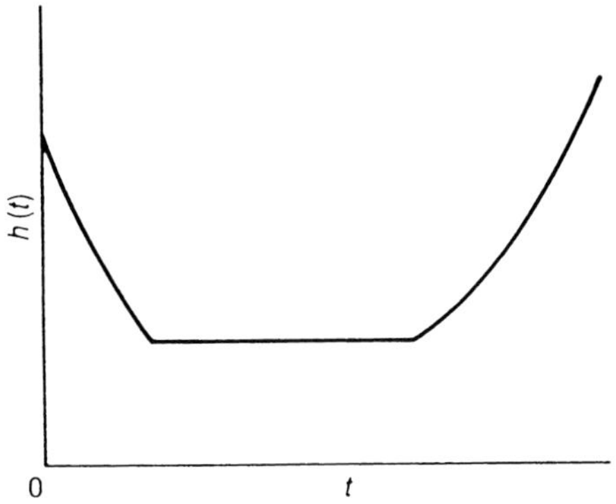

Fig 6 Bathtub curve: shape of hazard function for death in humans.

Bayesian confidence interval: An interval of a *posterior distribution* which is such that the density at any point inside the interval is greater than the density at any point outside. For any probability level, there is generally only one such interval, which is also often known as the *highest posterior density region.*

Bayesian inference: Statistical inference based on *Bayes' theorem.* The focus of the Bayesian approach is the *probability distribution* of any unknowns, given available information. In particular, the process deals with probabilities of hypotheses and probability distributions of parameters, neither of which feature in classical statistical inference. If, for example, interest centres on the hypothesis that two treatment means are equal, the result of a Bayesian test is the probability that the means are equal, given the data. In addition, the probability that the difference between treatment means is contained in any interval can be calculated to give a *Bayesian confidence interval.*

Bayes' theorem: A procedure for revising and updating the probability of some event in the light of new evidence. In its simplest form, the theorem may be written in terms of *conditional probabilities* as

$$P(A|B) = \frac{P(B|A)P(A)}{P(B)}$$

where $P(A|B)$ denotes the conditional probability of event A conditional on event B. The updated probability of the event after receiving new information is called the *posterior probability*. The theorem originates in an essay by the Reverend Thomas Bayes, published in 1763. To put the theorem into a medical context, suppose, for example, that the event of interest (A) is that a patient has a particular disease, and that the conditioning event (B) is a positive result on a relevant diagnostic test. The *prevalence* of A gives the unconditional probability of the disease, $P(A)$. The *sensitivity* of the test gives the conditional probability of a positive result amongst patients with the disease, $P(B|A)$. The *specificity* of the test gives the conditional probability of a negative result amongst patients who are disease free, $P(\bar{B}|\bar{A})$ (using a 'bar' notation to indicate a negative result or disease free condition). The unconditional probability of a positive result on the test, $P(B)$ is obtained from

$$\begin{aligned} P(B) &= P(B|A)P(A) + P(B|\bar{A})P(\bar{A}) \\ &= \text{sensitivity} \times \text{prevalence} + (1 - \text{specificity}) \times (1 - \text{prevalence}) \end{aligned}$$

and so the theorem can now be put in the form

$$\text{P(disease|test positive)} = \frac{\text{sensitivity} \times \text{prevalence}}{\text{sensitivity} \times \text{prevalence} + (1 - \text{specificity}) \times (1 - \text{prevalence})}$$

Behrens–Fisher problem: The problem of testing for the equality of the means of two *normal distributions* that do not have the same variance. Various *test statistics* have been proposed, although none are completely satisfactory. The one that is most commonly used, however, is given by

$$t = \frac{\bar{x}_1 - \bar{x}_2}{\sqrt{\frac{s_1^2}{n_1} + \frac{s_2^2}{n_2}}}$$

where $\bar{x}_1, \bar{x}_2, s_1^2, s_2^2, n_1$ and n_2 are the means, variances and sizes of samples of observations from each population. Under the hypothesis that the population means are equal, t has a *Student's t distribution* with ν degrees of freedom, where

$$\nu = \left[\frac{c^2}{n_1 - 1} + \frac{(1-c)^2}{n_2 - 1}\right]^{-1}$$

and

$$c = \frac{s_1^2/n_1}{s_1^2/n_1 + s_2^2/n_2}$$

See also **Welch's statistic**.

Believe the negative rule: See **believe the positive rule**.

Believe the positive rule: A rule for combining two *diagnostic tests*, A and B, in which 'disease present' is the diagnosis given if either A or B or both are positive. An alternative *believe the negative rule* assigns a patient to the disease class only if both A and B are positive. These rules do not necessarily have better *positive predictive values* than a single test; whether they do depends on the association between test outcomes.

Bellman–Harris process: A process evolving from an initial individual, in which each individual lives for a random length of time and at the end of its life produces a random number of offspring of the same type.

Bell-shaped distribution: A *probability distribution* having the overall shape of a vertical cross-section of a bell. The *normal distribution* is the most well-known example, but *Student's t-distribution* is also this shape.

Benchmarking: A procedure for adjusting a less reliable series of observations to make it consistent with more reliable measurements or *benchmarks*. For example, data on hospital bed occupation collected monthly will not necessarily agree with figures collected annually, and the monthly figures (which are likely to be less reliable) may be adjusted at some point to agree with the more reliable annual figures.

Benchmarks: See **benchmarking**.

Berkson's fallacy: The existence of artifactual correlations between diseases or between a disease and a *risk factor*, arising from the interplay of differential admission rates from an underlying population to a select study group, such as a series of hospital admissions. In any study that purports to establish an association, and where it appears likely that differential rates of admission apply, then at least some portion of the observed association should be suspect as attributable to this phenomenon.

Bernoulli distribution: The *probability distribution* of a *binary variable*, x, where $P(x = 1) = p$ and $P(x = 0) = 1 - p$.

Best linear unbiased estimator (BLUE): A *linear estimator* of a parameter that has smaller variance than any similar estimator of the parameter.

Beta-binomial distribution: The *probability distribution* obtained by averaging the parameter, p, of a *binomial distribution* over a *beta distribution*. Also known as a *Polyá distribution*.

Beta coefficient: A *regression coefficient* that is standardized so as to allow for a direct comparison between explanatory variables as to their relative explanatory power for the response variable. Calculated from the raw regression coefficients by multiplying them by the standard deviation of the corresponding explanatory variable.

Beta distribution: The *probability distribution* given by

$$f(x) = \frac{\Gamma(\alpha+\beta)}{\Gamma(\alpha)\Gamma(\beta)} x^{\alpha-1}(1-x)^{\beta-1}, \quad 0 < x < 1$$

where Γ is the *gamma function*. The mean of the distribution is $\alpha/(\alpha+\beta)$ and its variance is $\alpha\beta/[(\alpha+\beta)^2(\alpha+\beta+1)]$.

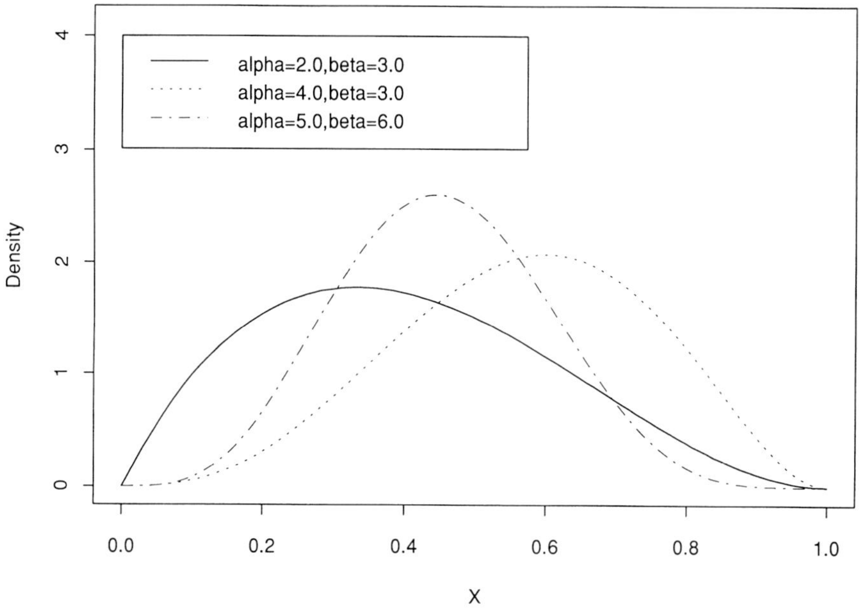

Fig 7 Beta distributions for a number of parameter values.

Beta(β)-error: Synonym for **type II error**.

Beta-geometric distribution: A *probability distribution* arising from assuming that the parameter, p, of a *geometric distribution* has itself a *beta distribution*. The distribution has been used to model the number of menstrual cycles required to achieve pregnancy.

Between groups matrix of sums of squares and cross products: See **multivariate analysis of variance**.

Between groups mean square: See **mean squares**.

Between groups sum of squares: See **analysis of variance**.

Bezugsiffer: The equivalent number of person-lifetimes at risk in a sample of varying ages; used to estimate the lifetime risk of a disease in a population.

Bias: Deviation of results or inferences from the truth, or processes leading to such deviation. More specifically, the extent to which the statistical method used in a study does not estimate the quantity thought to be estimated, or does not test the hypothesis to be tested. In estimation, a more precise definition is that an estimator $\hat{\theta}$ of a parameter θ is biased if $E(\hat{\theta}) \neq \theta$, where E denotes *expected value*. An estimator for which $E(\hat{\theta}) = \theta$ is said to be *unbiased*. See also **ascertainment bias, recall bias** and **selection bias**.

Biased coin method: A method of *random allocation* sometimes used in *clinical trials* in an attempt to avoid major inequalities in treatment numbers. At each point in the trial, the treatment with the fewest number of patients thus far is assigned a probability greater than a half of being allocated, the next patient. If the two treatments have equal numbers of patients, then simple randomization is used for the next patient.

Bimodal distribution: A *probability distribution*, or a *frequency distribution*, with two modes.

Binary sequence: A sequence whose elements take one of only two possible values, usually denoted 0 or 1. See also **Bernoulli distribution** and **binomial distribution**.

Binary variable: Observations which occur in one of two possible states, these often being labelled 0 and 1. Such data is frequently encountered in medical investigations; commonly occurring examples include 'dead/alive', 'improved/not improved' and 'depressed/not depressed'. Data involving this type of variable often require specialized techniques such as *logistic regression* for their analysis. See also **Bernoulli distribution**.

Binomial distribution: The *probability distribution* of the number of 'successes', x, in a series of n independent trials, each of which can result in either a 'success' or a 'failure'. The probability of a success, p, remains constant from trial to trial. Specifically, the distribution of x is given by

$$P(x) = \frac{n!}{x!(n-x)!}p^x(1-p)^{n-x}, \quad x = 0, 1, 2, \cdots, n$$

The mean of the distribution is np and its variance is $np(1-p)$.

Binomial index of dispersion: An index used to test whether k samples come from populations having *binomial distributions* with the same parameter p. Specifically, the index is calculated as

$$\sum_{i=1}^{k} n_i(P_i - P)^2/[P(1-P)]$$

where $n_1, n_2, \cdots, n_k$ are the respective sample sizes, $P_1, P_2, \cdots, P_k$ are the separate sample estimates of the probability of a 'success', and P is the mean proportion of successes taken over all samples. If the samples are all from a binomial distribution with parameter p, the index has a *chi-squared distribution* with $k - 1$ degrees of freedom. See also **index of dispersion**.

Bioassay: The process of evaluating the potency of a stimulus by analysing the response it produces in biological organisms. Examples of a stimulus in this context are a drug, a hormone, radiation and an environmental effect. See also **probit analysis**.

Bioavailability: The study of the variables which influence and determine the amount of active drug which gets from the administered dose to the site of pharmacologic action, as well as the rate at which it gets there.

Bioequivalence: The degree to which clinically important outcomes of treatment by a new preparation resemble those of a previously established preparation.

Bioequivalence trials: Trials carried out to compare two or more formulations of a drug containing the same active ingredient, in order to determine whether the different formulations give rise to comparable blood levels.

Biological assay: Synonym for **bioassay**.

Biological efficacy: The effect of treatment for all persons who receive the therapeutic agent to which they were assigned. It measures the biologic action of treatment among compliant persons.

Biostatistics: The branch of science which applies statistical methods to biological problems.

Biplots: A graphical display of *multivariate data* designed to show any structure or pattern amongst the individuals, for example, groups of similar individuals, or *outliers*; and in addition to display the relationships between variables. (See Fig. 8.) See also **principal components analysis**.

Bipolar factor: A factor, resulting from the application of *factor analysis*, which has a mixture of positive and negative loadings. Such factors can be difficult to interpret, and attempts are often made to simplify them by the process of *factor rotation*.

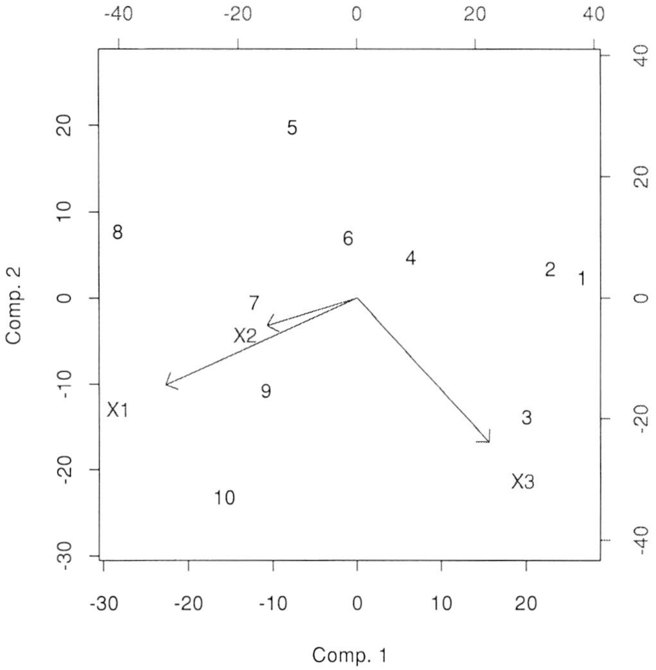

Fig 8 Biplot of a set of three-dimensional data.

Birth-cohort study: A *prospective study* of people born in a defined period.

Birth–death process: A *stochastic process* concerned with population changes due to births, deaths, immigration and emigration.

Birth–death ratio: The ratio of number of births to number of deaths within a given time in a population.

Birth order: The ranking of siblings according to age, starting with the eldest in the family.

Birth rate: The number of births occurring in a region in a given time period, divided by the size of the population of the region at the middle of the time period, usually expressed per 1000 population. For example, the birth rates for a number of countries in 1966 were as follows:

Country	Birth rate/1000
Egypt	42.1
India	20.9
Japan	17.3
Canada	24.8
USA	21.7

Birthweight: Infant's weight recorded at the time of birth. Low birthweight is defined to be values below 2500g, and very low birthweight, values below 1500g.

Biserial correlation: A measure of the strength of the relationship between two variables, one continuous (y) and the other recorded as a *binary variable* (x), but having underlying continuity and normality. Estimated from the sample values as

$$r_b = \frac{\bar{y}_1 - \bar{y}_0}{s_y} \frac{pq}{u}$$

where $\bar{y}_1$ is the sample mean of the y variable for those individuals for whom $x = 1$, $\bar{y}_0$ is the sample mean of the y variable for those individuals for whom $x = 0$, s_y is the standard deviation of the y values, p is the proportion of individuals with $x = 1$, and $q = 1 - p$ is the proportion of individuals with $x = 0$. Finally u is the ordinate (height) of the *standard normal distribution* at the point of division between the p and q proportions of the curve. See also **point-biserial correlation**.

Bit: A unit of information, consisting of one binary digit.

Bivariate data: Data in which the subjects each have measurements on two variables.

Bivariate distribution: The *joint distribution* of two *random variables*, x and y. A well-known example is the *bivariate normal distribution*, which has the form

$$f(x,y) = \frac{1}{2\pi\sigma_1\sigma_2\sqrt{1-\rho^2}} \times \exp\left\{-\frac{1}{1-\rho^2}\left[\frac{(x-\mu_1)^2}{\sigma_1^2} - 2\rho\frac{(x-\mu_1)(y-\mu_2)}{\sigma_1\sigma_2} + \frac{(y-\mu_2)^2}{\sigma_2^2}\right]\right\}$$

where $\mu_1, \mu_2, \sigma_1, \sigma_2, \rho$ are, respectively, the means, standard deviations and correlation of the two variables.

Bivariate normal distribution: See **bivariate distribution**.

Bivariate Oja median: An alternative to the more common *spatial median* as a measure of location for *bivariate data*. Defined as the value of θ that minimizes the objective function, $T(\theta)$, given by

$$T(\theta) = \sum_{i<j} A(\mathbf{x}_i, \mathbf{x}_j, \theta)$$

where $A(a, b, c)$ is the area of the triangle with vertices a, b, c, and $\mathbf{x}_1, \mathbf{x}_2, \cdots, \mathbf{x}_n$ are n bivariate observations.

Bivariate survival data: Data in which two related *survival times* are of interest. For example, in familial studies of disease *incidence*, data may be available on the ages and causes of death of fathers and their sons.

Blinding: A procedure used in *clinical trials* to avoid the possible *bias* that might be introduced if the patient and/or doctor knew which treatment the patient would be receiving. If neither the patient nor the doctor is aware of which treatment has been given, the trial is termed *double-blind*. If only one of the patient or doctor is unaware, the trial is called *single-blind*. Clinical trials should use the maximum degree of blindness that is possible, although in some areas, for example, surgery, it is often impossible for an investigation to be double-blind.

Block: A term used in experimental design to refer to a homogeneous grouping of experimental units (often subjects) designed to enable the experimenter to isolate and, if necessary, eliminate, variability due to extraneous causes. See also **randomized block design**.

Block randomization: A *random allocation* procedure used to keep the numbers of subjects in the different groups of a *clinical trial* closely balanced at all times. For example, if subjects are considered in sets of four at a time, there are six ways in which two treatments (A and B) can be allocated so that two subjects receive A and two receive B, namely

1. $AABB$	4. $BBAA$
2. $ABAB$	5. $BABA$
3. $ABBA$	6. $BAAB$

If only these six combinations are used for allocating treatments to each block of four subjects, the numbers in the two treatment groups can never, at any time, differ by more than two. See also **biased coin method** and **minimization**.

BLUE: Abbreviation for **best linear unbiased estimator**.

BMDP: A large and powerful statistical software package that allows the routine application of many statistical methods, including *Student's t-tests*, *regression analysis*, *factor analysis*, and *analysis of variance*. Modules for data entry and data management are also available, and the package is supported by a number of well-written manuals.

Body mass index: See **Quetelet's index**.

Bonferroni correction: A procedure for guarding against an increase in the *type I error* when performing multiple significance tests. To maintain the type I error at some selected value α, each of the m tests to be performed is judged against a *significance level*, α/m. For a small number of simultaneous tests (up to five), this method provides a simple and acceptable answer to the problem of multiple testing. It is, however, highly conservative and not recommended if large numbers of tests are to be applied, when one of the many other *multiple comparison tests* available is generally preferable. See also **least significant difference test** and **Newman–Keuls test**.

Bootstrap: A data-based *simulation* method for statistical inference, which can be used to study the variability of estimated characteristics of the *probability distribution* of a set of observations, and provide *confidence intervals* for parameters in situations where these are difficult or impossible to derive in the usual way. (The use of the term bootstrap derives from the phrase 'to pull oneself up by one's bootstraps'.) The basic idea of the procedure involves *sampling with replacement* to produce random samples of size n from the original data, $x_1, x_2, \cdots, x_n$; each of these is known as a *bootstrap sample* and each provides an estimate of the parameter of interest. Repeating the process a large number of times provides the required information on the variability of the estimator, and an approximate 95% confidence interval can, for example, be derived from the 2.5% and 97.5% *quantiles* of the replicate values. See also **jackknife**.

Bootstrap samples: See **bootstrap**.

Borrowing effect: A term used when abnormally low *standardized mortality rates* for one or more causes of death may be a reflection of an increase in the *proportional mortality rates* for other causes of death. For example, in a study of vinyl chloride workers, the overall proportional mortality rate for cancer indicated approximately a 50% excess, as compared with cancer death rates in the male US population. (One interpretation of this is a possible deficit of non-cancer deaths due to the *healthy worker effect*). Because the overall proportional mortality rate must by definition be equal to unity, a deficit in one type of mortality must entail a 'borrowing' from other causes.

Bowker's test for symmetry: A test that can be applied to *square contingency tables*, to assess the hypothesis that the probability of being in cell i, j is equal to the probability of being in cell j, i. Under this hypothesis, the *expected frequencies* in both cells are $(n_{ij} + n_{ji})/2$, where n_{ij} and n_{ji} are the corresponding observed frequencies. The *test statistic* is

$$X^2 = \sum_{i<j} \frac{(n_{ij} - n_{ji})^2}{n_{ij} + n_{ji}}$$

Under the hypothesis of symmetry, X^2 has approximately a *chi-squared distribution* with $c(c-1)/2$ degrees of freedom, where c is the number of rows of the table (and the number of columns). In the case of a *two-by-two contingency table*, the procedure is equivalent to *McNemar's test.*

Box-and-whisker plot: A graphical method of displaying the important characteristics of a set of observations. The display is based on the *five-number summary* of the data, with the 'box' part covering the *inter-quartile range*, and the 'whiskers' extending to include all but *outside observations*, these being indicated separately.

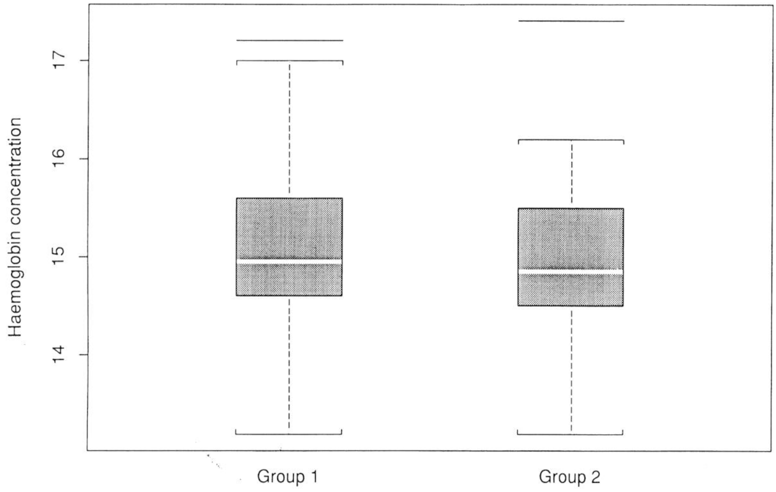

Fig 9 Box-and-whisker plot of haemoglobin concentrations for two groups of men.

Box–Cox transformation: A family of data transformations designed to achieve normality and given by

$$y = (x^\lambda - 1)/\lambda, \qquad \lambda \neq 0$$
$$y = \ln x, \qquad \lambda = 0$$

Maximum likelihood estimation can be used to estimate a suitable value of λ for a particular variable. See also **Taylor's power law**.

Box–Jenkins models: Synonym for **autoregressive moving average models**.

Box–Müller transformation: A method of generating *random variables* from a *normal distribution* by using variables from a *uniform distribution* in the interval (0,1). Specifically, if U_1 and U_2 are random uniform (0,1) variates, then

$$X = (-2 \ln U_1)^{\frac{1}{2}} \cos 2\pi U_2$$
$$Y = (-2 \ln U_1)^{\frac{1}{2}} \sin 2\pi U_2$$

are independent *standard normal variables*. Often used for generating data from a normal distribution when using *simulation*.

Box–Pierce test: A test to determine whether *time series* data are simply a *white noise sequence* and that therefore the observations are not related. The *test statistic* is

$$Q_m = n(n+2)\sum_{k=1}^{m} r_k^2/(n-k)$$

where r_k, $k = 1, 2, \cdots, m$, are the values of the *autocorrelations* up to lag m, and n is the number of observations in the series. If the data are a white noise series, then Q_m has a *chi-squared distribution* with m degrees of freedom. The test is valid only if m is very much less than n.

Box plot: Synonym for **box-and-whisker plot**.

Box's test: A test for assessing the equality of the variances in a number of populations that is less sensitive to departures from normality than *Bartlett's test*. See also **Hartley's test**.

Branch-and-bound algorithm: Synonym for **leaps-and-bounds algorithm**.

Branching process: A *stochastic process* in which individuals give rise to offspring, the distribution of descendents being likened to branches of a family tree.

Breakdown point: A measure of the insensitivity of an estimator to multiple *outliers* in the data. Roughly, it is given by the smallest fraction of data contamination needed to cause an arbitrarily large change in the estimate.

Brown–Forsythe test: A procedure for assessing whether a set of population variances are equal, based on applying an *F-test* to the following values calculated for a sample of observations from each of the populations:

$$z_{ij} = |x_{ij} - m_i|$$

where x_{ij} is the jth observation in the ith group and m_i is the median of the ith group. See also **Box's test**, **Bartlett's test** and **Hartley's test**.

Brownian motion: A continuous-time, continuous-state *stochastic process*, $\{x_t;\ t > 0\}$, for which: (1) $x_t - x_0$ has a *normal distribution* with mean μt and variance $\sigma^2 t$, where μ is known as the *drift parameter*; (2) all non-overlapping increments, $x_{t_1} - x_{t_0}, x_{t_2} - x_{t_1}, \cdots, x_{t_n} - x_{t_{n-1}}$, where $0 \leq t_0 \leq t_1, \cdots, \leq t_n$, are independent *random variables*. Brownian motion is the analog, in continuous time of sums of independent random variables.

Brushing scatterplots: An interactive computer graphics technique sometimes useful for exploring *multivariate data*. All possible two-variable *scatterplots* are displayed, and the points falling in a defined area of one of them (the 'brush') are highlighted in all.

Bubble plot: A method for displaying observations which involve three variable values. Two of the variables are used to form a *scatter diagram* and values of the third variable are represented by circles with differing radii centered at the appropriate position.

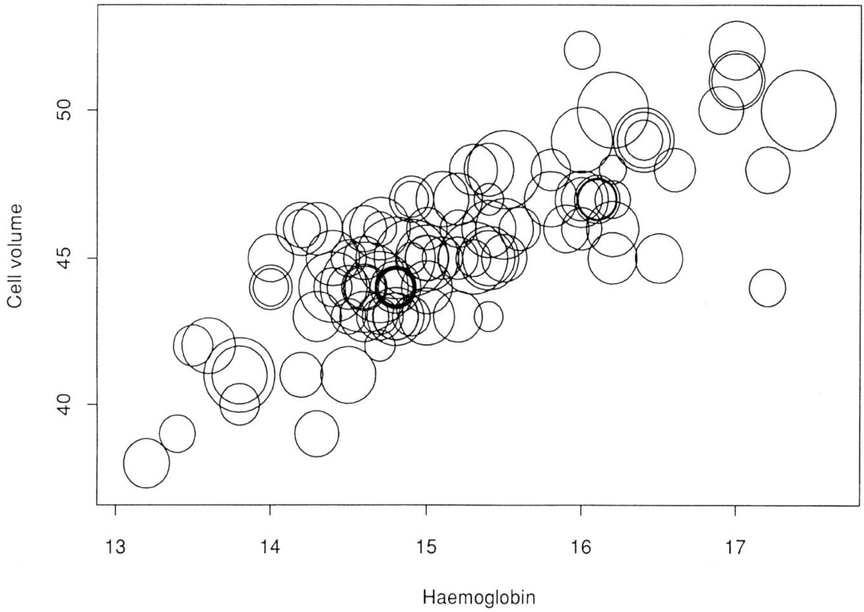

Fig 10 Bubble plot of haemoglobin concentration versus cell volume, with the radii of the circles proportional to the white blood count.

Bump hunting: A colourful term for the examination of *frequency distributions* for local maxima or modes that might be indicative of separate groups of subjects. See also **finite mixture distributions**.

Burgess method: See **point scoring**.

BW statistic: See **Cliff and Ord's BW statistic**.

Byte: A unit of information, as used in digital computers, equal to eight *bits*.

C

C: A high level programming language developed at Bell laboratories. Widely used for software development.

C++: A general purpose programming language which is a superset of *C*.

Calendarization: A generic term for *benchmarking*.

Calibration: A process that enables a series of easily obtainable but inaccurate measurements of some quantity of interest to be used to provide more precise estimates of the required values. Suppose, for example, there is a well-established, accurate method of measuring the concentration of a given chemical compound, but that it is too expensive and/or cumbersome for routine use. A cheap and easy to apply alternative is developed that is, however, known to be imprecise and possibly subject to *bias*. By using both methods over a range of concentrations of the compound, and applying *regression analysis* to the values from the cheap method and the corresponding values from the accurate method, a *calibration curve* can be constructed that may, in future applications, be used to read off estimates of the required concentration from the values given by the less involved, inaccurate method.

Calibration curve: See **calibration**.

California score: A score used in studies of sudden infant death syndrome that gives the number from eight adverse conditions present for a given infant. The events include: fewer than 11 antenatal visits; male sex; birthweight under 3000g and mother under 25 years old.

Caliper matching: See **matching**.

Canberra metric: A *dissimilarity coefficient* given by

$$d_{ij} = \sum_{k=1}^{q} |x_{ik} - x_{jk}|/(x_{ik} + x_{jk})$$

where $x_{ik}, x_{jk}, k = 1, \cdots, q$ are the observations on q variables for individuals i and j.

Canonical correlation analysis: A method of analysis for investigating the relationship between two groups of variables, by finding *linear functions* of one of the sets of variables that maximally correlate with linear functions of the variables in the other set. In many respects, the method can be viewed as an extension of *multiple regression* to situations involving more than a single response variable. Alternatively, it can be considered as analogous to *principal components analysis*, except that a correlation rather than a variance is maximized. A simple example of where this type of technique might be of interest is when the results of tests for, say, reading speed (x_1), reading power (x_2), arithmetical speed (y_1), and arithmetical power (y_2), are available from a sample of school children, and the question of interest is whether or not reading ability (measured by x_1 and x_2) is related to arithmetical ability (as measured by y_1 and y_2).

Canonical discriminant functions: See **discriminant analysis.**

Canonical variates: See **discriminant analysis.**

Capture–recapture sampling: A sampling scheme used in situations where the aim is to estimate the total number of individuals in a population. An initial sample is obtained and the individuals in that sample marked or otherwise identified. A second sample is, subsequently, independently obtained, and it is noted how many individuals in that sample are marked. If the second sample is representative of the population as a whole, then the sample proportion of marked individuals should be about the same as the corresponding population proportion. From this relationship, the total number of individuals in the population can be estimated. Specifically, if X individuals are 'captured', marked and released, and y individuals then independently captured, of which x are marked, then the estimator of population size (sometimes known as the *Petersen estimator*) is

$$\hat{N} = \frac{y}{x}X$$

with variance given by

$$\text{var}(\hat{N}) = \frac{Xy(X-x)(y-x)}{x^3}$$

Used originally to estimate the size of animal populations, the method is now also used to assess the size of many populations of great interest in medicine, for example, the number of drug users in a particular area and the completeness of cancer registry data.

Carryover effects: See **crossover design.**

CART: Abbreviation for **classification and regression tree technique.**

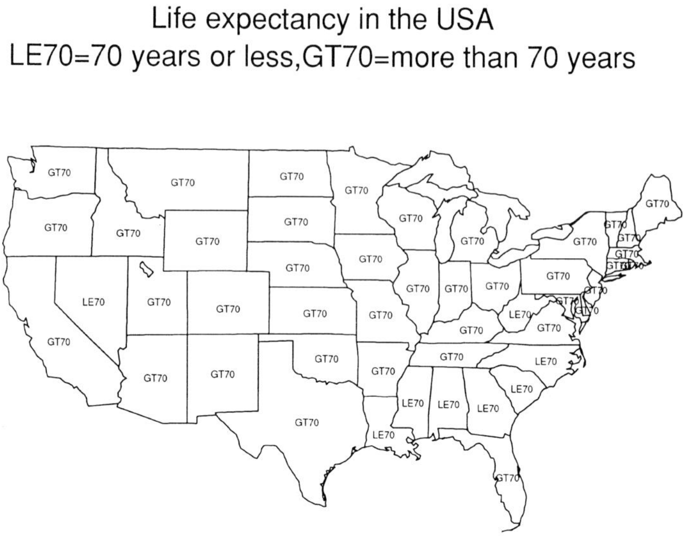

Fig 11 Cartogram of life expectancy in the USA.

Cartogram: A diagram in which descriptive statistical information is displayed on a geographical map by means of shading or by using a variety of different symbols.

Case: A term most often used in *epidemiology* for a person in the population or study group identified as having the disease or condition of interest.

Case–control study: See **retrospective study**.

Case-crossover design: A procedure for the analysis of transient effects on the risk of acute illness events. The idea behind the method is to ask a patient whether he or she was engaged in some activity or exposed to a suspected cause immediately before the event, and to compare the response to the 'usual' frequency with which he or she engages in the activity or is exposed. In this way each case is its own control. The hypothesis that vigorous exercise predisposes to heart attacks, for example, might be investigated by such a design with cases being asked about their usual frequency of taking vigorous exercise and about whether they were engaged in such activity immediately before their heart attack.

Case-fatality rate: The probability of death amongst diagnosed cases of a disease. Specifically defined as number of deaths due to the disease in a specified time period divided by the number of cases of the disease at the beginning of the period. Typically used in acute infectious diseases such as AIDS.

Case-heterogeneity study: A procedure for the estimation of *relative risks*, not against a set of non-diseased population referents, but against a set of subjects with other diseases, some of which may also have an association with the same exposure factors or their correlates.

Catalytic epidemic models: Models concerned with the age distribution at attack of infectious disease. The simplest such model assumes that a constant force of infection acts upon members of a susceptible population. More generally, the force of infection is allowed to be a function of the age of a susceptible individual.

Categorical variable: A variable that gives the appropriate label of an observation after allocation to one of several possible categories, for example, gender: male or female, marital status: married, single or divorced, or blood group: A, B, AB or O. The categories are often given numerical labels, but for this type of data these have no numerical significance. See also **binary variable, continuous variable** and **ordinal variable**.

Causality: The relating of causes to the effects they produce. Many investigations in medicine seek to establish causal links between events, for example, that receiving treatment A causes patients to live longer than taking treatment B. In general, the strongest claims to have established causality come from data collected in *experimental studies*. Relationships established in *observational studies* may be very suggestive of a causal link, but are always open to alternative explanations.

Causal risk difference: The difference between the rate of disease that would have been observed if the entire study population had been exposed, and the rate of disease that would have been observed if the entire study population had been unexposed.

Cause-specific death rate: A death rate calculated for people dying from a particular disease. For example, the following are the rates per 1000 people for three disease classes for developed and developing countries in 1985.

	C1	C2	C3
Developed	0.5	4.5	2.0
Developing	4.5	1.5	0.6

C1 = Infectious and parasitic diseases
C2 = Circulatory diseases
C3 = Cancer

See also **crude death rate** and **age-specific death rate**.

Ceiling effect: A term used to describe what happens when many subjects in a study have scores on a variable that are at or near the possible upper limit ('ceiling'). Such an effect may cause problems for some types of analysis, because it reduces the possible amount of variation in the variable. The converse, or *floor effect*, causes similar problems.

Cellular proliferation models: Models used to describe the growth of cell populations. One example is the *deterministic* model

$$N(t) = N(t_0)e^{\nu(t-t_0)}$$

where $N(t)$ is the number of cells in the population at time t, t_0 is an initial time and ν represents the difference between a constant birth rate and a constant death rate. Often also viewed as a *stochastic process* in which $N(t)$ is considered to be a *random variable*.

Censored observations: An observation x_i is said to be censored if it is known that, given L_i and U_i, the exact value of x_i is unknown, only that $x_i \leq U_i$ or $x_i \geq L_i$. Such observations arise most frequently in studies where the main response variable is time until a particular event occurs (for example, time to death) when at the completion of the study, the event of interest has not happened to a number of subjects. See also **interval censored data, singly censored observations, doubly censored data** and **non-informative censoring**.

Census: A study that involves the observation of every member of a population.

Centile: Synonym for **percentile**.

Centile reference charts: Charts used in medicine to observe clinical measurements on individual patients in the context of population values. If the population *centile* corresponding to the subject's value is atypical, this may indicate an underlying pathological condition. The chart can also provide a background with which to compare the measurement as it changes over time. (See Fig. 12 opposite.)

Centralized database: A *database* held and maintained in a central location, particularly in a *multicentre study*.

Central limit theorem: If a *random variable* y has population mean μ and population variance σ^2, then the sample mean, $\bar{y}$, based on n observations, has an approximate *normal distribution* with mean μ and variance σ^2/n, for sufficiently large n.

Central range: The range within which the central 90% of values of a set of observations lie.

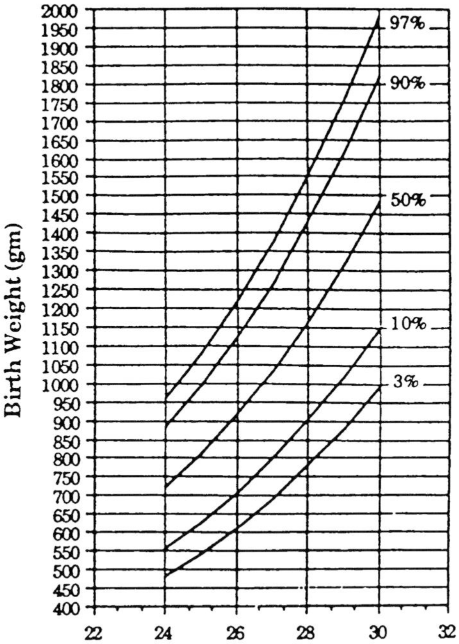

Fig 12 Centile chart of birthweight for gestational age.

Central tendency: A property of the distribution of a variable, usually measured by statistics such as the mean, median and mode.

CFA: Abbreviation for **confirmatory factor analysis**.

Chain-binomial models: Models arising in the mathematical theory of infectious diseases, that postulate that at any stage in an epidemic there are a certain number of infected and susceptibles, and that it is reasonable to suppose that the latter will yield a fresh crop of cases at the next stage, the number of new cases having a *binomial distribution*. This results in a 'chain' of binomial distributions, the actual probability of a new infection at any stage depending on the numbers of infectives and susceptibles at the previous stage.

Chaining: A phenomenon often encountered in the application of *single linkage clustering*, which relates to the tendency of the method to incorporate intermediate points between distinct clusters into an existing cluster rather than initiate a new one.

Chains of infection: A description of the course of an infection amongst a set of individuals. The susceptibles infected by direct contact with the introductory cases are said to make up the first generation of cases; the susceptibles infected by direct contact with the first generation are said to make up the second generation and so on. The enumeration of the number of cases in each generation is called an *epidemic chain*. Thus the sequence 1-2-1-0 denotes a chain consisting of one introductory case, two first generation cases, one second generation case and no cases in later generations.

Change point models: Models for the relationship between two variables in situations where some change in the relationship might have occured at a particular time point. A very simple example of such a model is the following;

$$y_i = \alpha_1 + \beta_1 x_i + e_i, \;\; i = 1, \cdots, \tau$$
$$y_i = \alpha_2 + \beta_2 x_i + e_i, \;\; i = \tau + 1, \cdots, T$$

Interest would centre on estimating the parameters in the model, particularly the change point, τ.

Change scores: Scores obtained by subtracting a post-treatment score on some variable from the corresponding pre-treatment, baseline value. See also **adjusting for baseline** and **baseline balance**.

Chaos: Apparently random behaviour exhibited by data generated from a *deterministic model.*

Chapman–Kolmogorov equations: A set of equations used in the theory of *stochastic processes*, giving the state of a system at a certain time in terms of the known states at previous times.

Characteristic root: Synonym for **eigenvalue**.

Characteristic vector: Synonym for **eigenvector**.

Chebyshev's inequality: A statement about the proportion of observations that fall within some number of standard deviations of the mean for any *probability distribution*. One version is that for a *random variable*, x,

$$\text{Prob}\left[-k \leq \frac{x-\mu}{\sigma} \leq k\right] \leq 1 - \frac{1}{k^2}$$

where k is the number of standard deviations, σ, from the mean, μ. For example, the inequality states that at least 75% of the observations fall within two standard deviations of the mean. If the variable x can take on only positive values, then the following, known as the *Markov inequality*, holds:

$$\text{Prob}[x \leq X] \leq 1 - \frac{\mu}{X}$$

Chernoff's faces: A technique for representing *multivariate data* graphically. Each observation is represented by a computer generated face, the features of

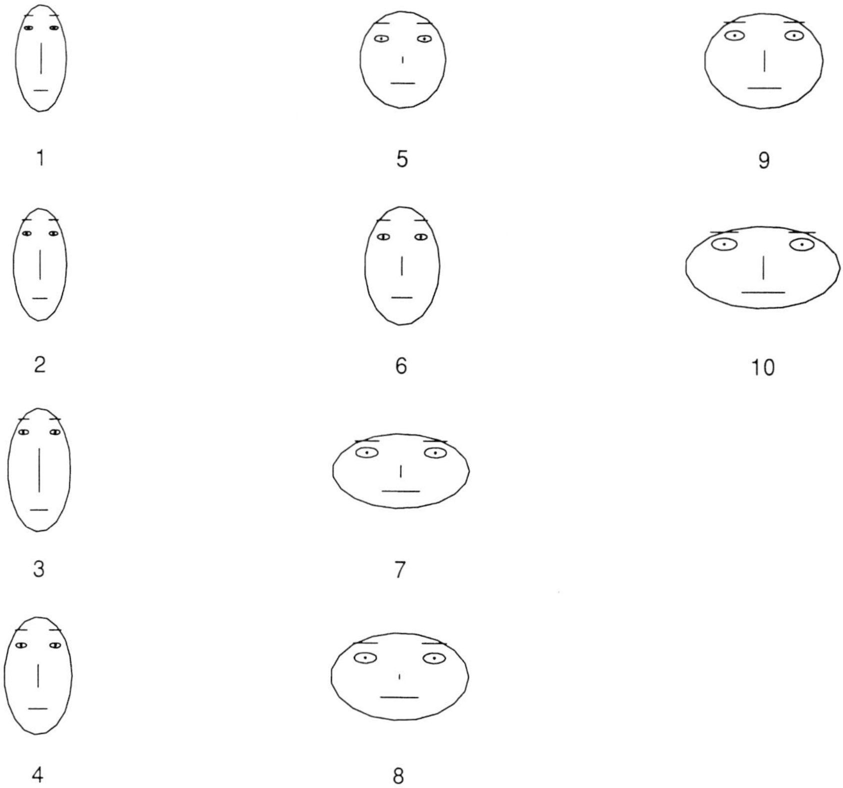

Fig 13 Chernoff's faces representing ten multivariate observations.

which are controlled by an observation's variable values. The collection of faces representing the set of observations may be useful in identifying groups of similar individuals, *outliers*, etc. See also **Andrews' plots** and **glyphs**.

Child death rate: The number of deaths of children aged one to four years in a given year per 1000 children in this age group.

Chi-squared distribution: The *probability distribution* of the sum of squares of a number (ν) of independent *standard normal variables*. The mathematical formula of the distribution is

$$f(x) = \frac{1}{2^{\nu/2}\Gamma(\nu/2)} x^{(\nu-2)/2} e^{-x/2}, \quad x > 0$$

i.e., a *gamma distribution* with $\alpha = \nu/2$. The parameter ν is usually known as the degrees of freedom of the distribution. This distribution arises in many areas of statistics, for example, assessing the *goodness-of-fit* of models, particularly those fitted to *contingency tables*.

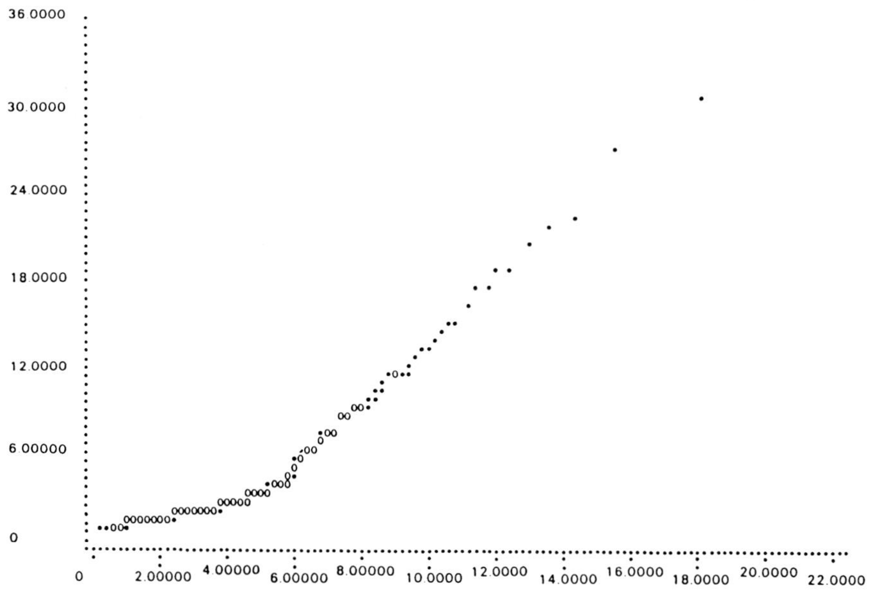

Fig 14 Chi-squared probability plot that indicates that these data do not have a multivariate normal distribution.

Chi-squared probability plot: A procedure for testing whether a set of *multivariate data* have a *multivariate normal distribution.* The ordered generalized distances

$$d_{(i)} = (\mathbf{x}_i - \bar{\mathbf{x}})'\mathbf{S}^{-1}(\mathbf{x}_i - \bar{\mathbf{x}})$$

where $\mathbf{x}_i, i = 1, \cdots, n$, are multivariate observations involving q variables, $\bar{\mathbf{x}}$ is the sample mean vector and $\mathbf{S}$ the sample *variance–covariance matrix*, are plotted against the *quantiles* of a *chi-squared distribution* with q degrees of freedom. Deviations from multivariate normality are indicated by depatures from a straight line in the plot. See also **quantile–quantile plot**.

Chi-squared statistic: A statistic having, at least approximately, a *chi-squared distribution.* An example is the *test statistic* used to assess the independence of the two variables forming a *contingency table* with r rows and c columns:

$$X^2 = \sum_{i=1}^{r}\sum_{j=1}^{c}(O_i - E_i)^2/E_i$$

where O_i represents an observed value and E_i the *expected frequency* under independence. Under the hypothesis of independence, X^2 has, approximately, a chi-squared distribution with $(r - 1)(c - 1)$ degrees of freedom.

Chi-squared test for trend: A test applied to a *two-dimensional contingency table* in which one variable has two categories and the other has k ordered categories, to assess whether there is a difference in the trend of the proportions in the two groups. The result of using the ordering in this way is a test that is more powerful than using the *chi-squared statistic* to test for independence.

Choleski decomposition: The decomposition of a *symmetric matrix*, $\mathbf{A}$, (which is not a *singular matrix*), into the form

$$\mathbf{A} = \mathbf{L}\mathbf{L}'$$

where $\mathbf{L}$ is a *lower triangular matrix.*

Circadian variation: The variation that takes place in variables such as blood pressure and body temperature over a 24 hour period.

City-block distance: A *distance measure* occasionally used in *cluster analysis* and given by

$$d_{ij} = \sum_{k=1}^{q} |x_{ik} - x_{jk}|$$

where q is the number of variables and $x_{ik}, x_{jk}, k = 1, \cdots, q$, are the observations on individuals i and j.

Class frequency: The number of observations in a class interval of the observed *frequency distribution* of a variable.

Classification and regression tree technique (CART): An alternative to *multiple regression* and associated techniques, for determining subsets of explanatory variables most important for the prediction of the response variable. Rather than fitting a model to the sample data, a *tree* structure is generated by dividing the sample recursively into a number of groups, each division being chosen so as to maximize some measure of the difference in the response variable in the resulting two groups. The resulting structure often provides easier interpretation than a regression equation, as those variables most important for prediction can be quickly identified. Additionally, this approach does not require distributional assumptions and is also more resistant to the effects of *outliers*. At each stage the sample is split on the basis of a single variable, x_i, or a set of variables, $x_1, x_2 \ldots x_q$, according to the answers to such questions as 'Is $x_i \leq c$' (univariate split), is '$\sum_{i=1}^{q} a_i x_i \leq c$' (*linear function* split) and 'does $x_i \in A$' (if x_i is a *categorical variable*). See also **automatic interaction detector**.

Classification matrix: A term often used in *discriminant analysis* for the matrix containing counts of correct classifications on the main diagonal and incorrect classifications elsewhere.

Classification rule: See **discriminant analysis.**

Classification techniques: A generic term used for both *cluster analysis* methods and *discriminant analysis*, although more widely applied to the former.

Classification tree: A statistical model for classification taking the form of a *tree*, the nodes of which split the set of subjects into subsets according to the values they have on a set of variables.

Class intervals: The intervals of the *frequency distribution* of a set of observations.

Clemmesen's hook: A phenomenon sometimes observed when interpreting parameter estimates from *age–period–cohort models*, where rates increase to some maximum, but then fall back slightly before continuing their upward trend.

Cliff and Ord's BW statistic: A measure of the degree to which the presence of some factor in an area (or time period) increases the chances that this factor will be found in a nearby area. Defined explicitly as

$$\text{BW} = \sum_i \sum_j \delta_{ij}(x_i - x_j)^2$$

where $x_i = 1$ if the ith area has the characteristic and zero otherwise, and $\delta_{ij} = 1$ if areas i and j are adjacent and zero otherwise. See also **Moran's I**.

Clinical decision analysis: A procedure designed to provide insight into the structure of a clinical problem and to identify the main determinants of diagnostic and therapeutic choice. The procedure has four distinct stages:

- defining the clinical problem and structuring it as a *decision tree*. This includes descriptions of the patient, of the possible diagnostic and therapeutic actions, and of the possible outcomes after treatment;
- estimating probabilities for diagnostic and therapeutic outcomes;
- performing the requisite computations for determining the preferred course of action;
- presentation of the results of the analysis in a clinically useful way.

Clinical priors: See **prior distribution**.

Clinical trial: A *prospective study* involving human subjects, designed to determine the effectiveness of a treatment, a surgical procedure, or a therapeutic regimen administered to patients with a specific disease.

Clinical trial simulator: A computer program that can be used to model real world *clinical trials*, and which is capable of rendering the implications of different designs and analysis decisions more tangible to individuals whose background and primary interests lie in medicine rather than statistics.

Clinical vs statistical significance: The distinction between results in terms of their possible clinical importance rather than simply in terms of their statistical significance. With large samples, for example, very small differences that have little or no clinical importance may turn out to be statistically significant. The practical implications of any finding in a medical investigation must be judged on clinical as well as statistical grounds.

Clinimetrics: The study of indices and rating scales used to describe or measure symptoms, physical signs and other clinical phenomena in clinical medicine.

Clonogenic assay: An assay designed to predict the chemosensitivity of a patient's tumour. A portion of the tumour is disaggregated and then planted in single-cell suspension. A proportion of the tumour cells divide and multiply into colonies that can be counted after a fixed time of growth. The inhibition of formation of these colonies by a chemotherapeutic agent suggests that this agent may also be of use in the treatment of the patient.

Closed and open birth interval data: The lengths of the 'closed' intervals from the ith to the $(i + 1)$th birth and of the 'open' intervals since the most recent birth for women who have had the same number of children. Considered useful indicators of current changes in natality patterns.

Closed sequential design: See **sequential analysis**.

CLUSTAN: A software package that implements many methods of *cluster analysis*, including *Ward's method*, *single linkage clustering* and *K-means cluster analysis*.

Cluster: See **disease cluster**.

Cluster analysis: A set of methods for constructing a (hopefully) sensible and informative classification of an initially unclassified set of data, using the variable values observed on each individual. See also **agglomerative hierarchical clustering, K-means cluster analysis**, and **finite mixture distribution**.

Clustered binary data: Data arising from observing *binary variables* in a *longitudinal study* or from subsampling of primary sampling units. Examples of the latter are common, for example, in opthalmology, where two eyes form a cluster but observations are taken on each eye, and in periodontology, where the mouth is the cluster but the data are gathered from multiple sites within the mouth. (In many cases the 'cluster' will be essentially the individual subject on whom several observations are made). A distinguishing feature of such data is that they tend to exhibit intracluster correlation, and their analysis needs to address this correlation to reach valid conclusions. Methods of analysis that ignore the correlations tend to be inadequate. In particular, they are likely to give estimates of standard errors that are too low. Suitable methods that can be used to analyze such data are the *mixed-effects logistic model* and the *generalized estimating equation* approach.

Cluster randomization: The *random allocation* of groups or clusters of individuals in the formation of treatment groups. Although not as statistically efficient as individual randomization, the procedure frequently offers important economic, feasibility or ethical advantages.

Cluster sampling: A method of sampling in which the members of a population are arranged in groups (the 'clusters'). A number of clusters are selected at random and those chosen are then subsampled. The clusters generally consist of natural groupings, for example, families, hospitals, schools, etc. See also **random sample, area sampling** and **quota sample**.

Cluster-specific models: Methods for the analysis of *clustered binary data* that model the response variable as a function of covariates and parameters specific to a particular cluster (in this context usually a subject). An example is the *mixed effects logistic model.* See also **population averaged models**.

C_{max}: A measure traditionally used to compare treatments in *bioequivalence studies.* The measure is simply the highest recorded response value for a subject. See also **area under curve** and $\mathbf{T_{max}}$.

Coale and Trussell model: A model for describing the variation in the age pattern of human fertility, which involves the product of terms representing natural fertility and fertility control.

Coarse data: A term sometimes used when the exact values in a data set are not observed. Examples include data containing *missing values* and data containing *censored observations.*

Cochran's C-test: A test that the variances of a number of populations are equal. The *test statistic* is

$$C = \frac{s_{\max}^2}{\sum_{i=1}^{g} s_i^2}$$

where g is the number of populations and $s_i^2, i = 1, \cdots, g$, are the variances of samples from each, of which $s_{\max}^2$ is the largest. Tables of *critical values* are available. See also **Bartlett's test, Box's test** and **Hartley's test**.

Cochran's Q-test: A procedure for assessing the hypothesis of no inter-observer *bias* in situations where a number of raters judge the presence or absence of some characteristic on a number of subjects. Essentially a generalized *McNemar's test*. The test statistic is given by

$$Q = \frac{r(r-1)\sum_{j=1}^{r}(y_{.j} - y_{..}/r)^2}{ry_{..} - \sum_{i=1}^{n} y_{i.}^2}$$

where $y_{ij} = 1$ if the ith patient is judged by the jth rater to have the characteristic present and 0 otherwise, $y_{i.}$ is the total number of raters who judge the ith subject to have the characteristic, $y_{.j}$ is the total number of subjects the jth rater judges as having the characteristic present, $y_{..}$ is the total number of 'present' judgements made, n is the number of subjects and r the number of raters. If the hypothesis of no inter-observer bias is true, Q has, approximately, a *chi-squared distribution* with $r - 1$ degrees of freedom.

Coefficient of alienation: A name sometimes used for $1 - r^2$, where r is the estimated value of the *correlation coefficient* of two *random* variables. See also **coefficient of determination.**

Coefficient of concordance: A coefficient used to assess the agreement among m raters ranking n individuals according to some specific characteristic. Calculated as

$$W = 12S/[m^2(n^3 - n)]$$

where S is the sum of squares of the differences between the total of the ranks assigned to each individual and the value $m(n+1)/2$. W can vary from 0 to 1 with the value 1 indicating perfect agreement.

Coefficient of determination: The square of the *correlation coefficient* between two variables. Gives the proportion of the variation in one variable that is accounted for by the other.

Coefficient of inbreeding: See **Wright's inbreeding coefficient**.

Coefficient of kinship: The probability that two homologous genes drawn at random, one from each of the two parents, will be identical and therefore homozygous in an offspring.

Coefficient of variation: A measure of spread for a set of data, defined as

$$100 \times \text{standard deviation/mean}$$

Originally proposed as a way of comparing the variability in different distributions, but found to be sensitive to errors in the mean.

Cohort: See **cohort study**.

Cohort study: An investigation in which a group of individuals (the *cohort*) is identified and followed prospectively, perhaps for many years, and their subsequent medical history recorded. The cohort may be subdivided at the onset into groups with different characteristics, for example, exposed and not exposed to some *risk factor*, and at some later stage a comparison made of the *incidence* of a particular disease in each group. See also **prospective study**.

Collapsing categories: A procedure often applied to *contingency tables* in which two or more row or column categories are combined, in many cases so as to yield a reduced table in which there are a larger number of observations in particular cells. Not to be recommended in general since it can lead to misleading conclusions. See also **Simpson's paradox**.

Collinearity: See **multicollinearity**.

Combination analysis: The analysis of *dose–response curves* of combinations of substances. Of particular importance when the effects of the combination differ from that expected from studying the single components administered alone. See also **synergism**.

Combination therapy trials: *Clinical trials* in which patients are treated with combinations of therapies. Such a trial would generally involve three ' treatments':

A and placebo
B and placebo
A and B

Two placebos are necessary in practice since it is unlikely that the two active treatments will be perfectly matched.

Commensurate variables: Variables that are on the same scale or expressed in the same units, for example, systolic and diastolic blood pressure.

Common factor: See **factor analysis**.

Common factor variance: A term used in *factor analysis* for that part of the variance of a variable shared with the other observed variables via the relationships of these variables to the *common factors*. Often known as *communality*.

Communality: See **common factor variance**.

Community controls: See **control group**.

Community intervention study: An *intervention study* in which the experimental unit to be randomized to different treatments is not an individual patient or subject but a group of people, for example, a school or a factory. See also **cluster randomization**.

COMPACT: A computer program for cancer trials which acts as an interface between the *clinical trial* data and standard statistical analysis packages.

Comparative bioavailability trial: A trial in which different formulations of a drug are administered to a number of subjects and blood samples obtained at various times following administration. Assay of the drug in the blood samples gives, for each administration of a formulation to a given subject, a sequence of concentrations of drug in the blood. The purpose of such trials is to assess the *in vivo* performances of the different formulations.

Comparative calibration: A term applied to the problem of comparing several distinct methods of measuring a given quantity.

Comparative exposure rate: A measure of association for use in a *matched case–control study*, defined as the ratio of the number of case–control pairs, where the case has greater exposure to the risk factor under investigation, to the number where the control has greater exposure. In simple cases the measure is equivalent to the *odds ratio* or a weighted combination of odds ratios. In more general cases the measure can be used to assess association when an odds ratio computation is not feasible.

Comparative trial: Synonym for **controlled trial**.

Comparison group: Synonym for **control group**.

Comparisonwise error rate: Synonym for **per-comparison error rate**.

Compartmental models: Models widely used in tracer kinetic studies to investigate the time course of a drug through some or all the stages of absorption, distribution, metabolism and elimination.

Competing risks: A term used particularly in the analysis of *survival times* to indicate that the event of interest (for example, death), may occur from more than one cause. For example, in a study of smoking as a *risk factor* for lung cancer, a subject who dies of coronary heart disease is no longer at risk of lung cancer. Consequently coronary heart disease is a competing risk in this situation.

Complementary log-log transformation: A transformation of a proportion, p, that is often a useful alternative to the *logistic transformation*. It is given by

$$y = \ln[-\ln(1-p)]$$

This function transforms a probability in the range (0,1) to a value in $(-\infty, \infty)$, but unlike the logistic and *probit transformation* it is not symmetric about the value $p = 0.5$. In the context of a *bioassay*, this transformation can be derived by supposing that the tolerances of individuals have a *Gumbel distribution*. Very similar to the logistic transformation when p is small.

Complete linkage cluster analysis: An *agglomerative hierarchical clustering method* in which the distance between two clusters is defined as the greatest distance between a member of one cluster and a member of the other.

Completely randomized design: An experimental design in which the treatments are allocated to the experimental units purely on a chance basis.

Complete spatial randomness: A *Poisson process* in the plane for which

- the number of events $N(A)$ in any region A follows a *Poisson distribution* with mean $\lambda|A|$,
- given $N(A) = n$, the events in A form an independent random sample from the uniform distribution on A.

Here $|A|$ denotes the area of A, and λ is the mean number of events per unit area. Often used as the standard against which to compare an observed spatial pattern.

Compliance: The extent to which patients in a *clinical trial* follow the trial *protocol.*

Component bar chart: A *bar chart* that shows the component parts of the aggregate represented by the total length of the bar. The component parts are shown as sectors of the bar with lengths in proportion to their relative size. Shading or colour can be used to enhance the display. (See Fig. 15.)

Composite hypothesis: A hypothesis that specifies more than a single value for a parameter. For example, the hypothesis that the mean of a population is greater than some value.

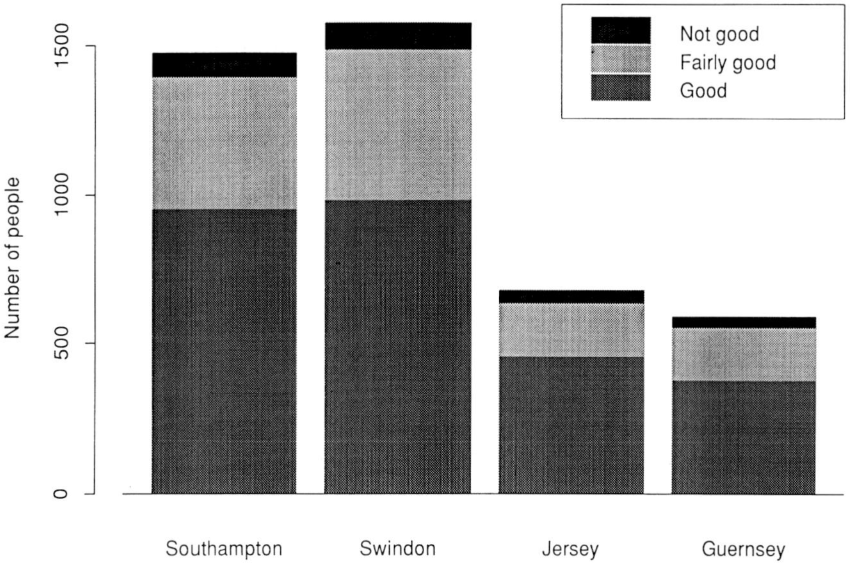

Fig 15 Component bar chart showing subjective health assessment in four regions.

Compositional data: A set of observations, $\mathbf{x}_1, \mathbf{x}_2, \cdots, \mathbf{x}_n$ for which each element of $\mathbf{x}_i$ is a proportion and the elements of $\mathbf{x}_i$ are constrained to sum to unity. For example, a number of blood samples might be analysed and the proportion, in each, of a number of chemical elements recorded.

Compound distribution: A type of *probability distribution* arising when the parameter of a distribution is itself a *random variable* with a corresponding probability distribution. For example, a *normal distribution* might be assigned to the *expected value* of a normal distribution. See also **contagious distribution**.

Compound symmetry: The property possessed by a *variance-covariance matrix* of a set of *multivariate data* when its main diagonal elements are equal to one another, and additionally its off-diagonal elements are also equal. Consequently, the matrix has the general form:

$$\Sigma = \begin{pmatrix} \sigma^2 & \rho\sigma^2 & \cdots & \rho\sigma^2 \\ \rho\sigma^2 & \sigma^2 & \cdots & \rho\sigma^2 \\ \vdots & \vdots & & \vdots \\ \rho\sigma^2 & \rho\sigma^2 & \cdots & \sigma^2 \end{pmatrix}$$

where ρ is the assumed common *correlation coefficient* of the measures. Of most importance in the analysis of *longitudinal data*. See also **Mauchly test**.

Computer-aided diagnosis: Computer programs designed to support clinical decision making. In general, such systems are based on the repeated application of *Bayes' theorem*. In some cases, a reasoning strategy is implemented that enables the programs to conduct clinically pertinent dialogue and explain their decisions. Such programs have been developed in a variety of diagnostic areas, for example, the diagnosis of dyspepsia and of acute abdominal pain. See also **expert system**.

Computer-assisted interviews: A method of interviewing subjects in which the interviewer reads the question from a computer screen instead of a printed page, and uses the keyboard to enter the answer. Skip patterns (i.e. 'if so-and-so, go to Question such-and-such') are built into the program, so that the screen automatically displays the appropriate question. Checks can be built in and an immediate warning given if a reply lies outside an acceptable range or is inconsistent with previous replies; revision of previous replies is permitted, with automatic return to the current question. The responses are entered directly on to the computer record, avoiding the need for subsequent coding and data entry. The program can make automatic selection of subjects who require additional procedures, such as special tests, supplementary questionnaires, or follow-up visits.

Computer virus: A computer program designed to sabotage by carrying out unwanted and often damaging operations. Viruses can be transmitted via discs or over *networks*. A number of procedures are available that provide protection against the problem.

Concentration measure: A measure, C, of the *dispersion* of a categorical *random variable*, Y, that assumes the integral values j, $1 \leq j \leq s$, with probability p_j, given by

$$C = 1 - \sum_{j=1}^{s} p_j^2$$

See also **entropy measure.**

Concomitant therapy: Other medication or treatment taken by the participants in a *clinical trial*, in addition to the trial treatment. If one of the experimental groups is receiving one or more of these additional therapies at a higher (or lower) rate than the others, it may complicate the interpretation of the study results.

Concomitant variables: Synonym for **covariates**.

Conditional distribution: The *probability distribution* of a *random variable* (or the *joint distribution* of several variables) when the values of one or more other random variables are held fixed.

Conditional independence graph: An *undirected graph* constructed so that if two variables, U and V, are connected only via a third variable W, then U and V are conditionally independent given W.

Conditional logistic regression: A form of *logistic regression* for use in a *matched case–control study*, in which the ratio of the *odds* of disease occurring in one member of a matched pair relative to the other member is modelled as

$$\ln\left\{\frac{p_1/(1-p_1)}{p_2(1-p_2)}\right\} = \beta_1(x_{11}-x_{21}) + \beta_2(x_{12}-x_{22}) + \cdots + \beta_q(x_{1q}-x_{2q})$$

where $x_{ij}, i=1,2; j=1,2,\cdots,q$ represent the values of q explanatory variables for the two individuals. The parameters in the model $(\beta_1, \beta_2, \cdots, \beta_q)$ are usually estimated by *maximum likelihood estimation*.

Conditional mortality rate: Synonym for **hazard function**.

Conditional probability: The probability that an event A occurs given the outcome of some other event, B. Usually written, $P(A|B)$. For example, the probability of a person being colour blind given that the person is male is about 0.1, and the corresponding probability given that the person is female is approximately 0.0001. It is not, of course, necessary that $P(A|B) = P(B|A)$; the probability of having spots given that a patient has measles, for example, is very high; the probability of measles given that a patient has spots is, however, much less. If $P(A|B) = P(A)$ then the events A and B are said to be independent. See also **Bayes' theorem**.

Confidence interval: A range of values, calculated from the sample observations, that are believed, with a particular probability, to contain the true parameter value. A 95% confidence interval, for example, implies that, were the estimation process repeated again and again, then 95% of the calculated intervals would be expected to contain the true parameter value. Note that the stated probability level refers to properties of the interval and not to the parameter itself, which is not considered a *random variable* (although, see **Bayesian inference**).

Confirmatory data analysis (CFA): A term often used for model fitting and inferential statistical procedures to distinguish them from the methods of *exploratory data analysis*.

Confirmatory factor analysis (CFA): See **factor analysis**.

Confounding: A process observed in some *factorial designs* in which it is impossible to differentiate between some *main effects* or *interactions*, on the basis of the particular design used. In essence, the *contrast* that measures one of the effects is exactly the same as the contrast that measures the other. The two effects are usually referred to as *aliases*.

Conservative and non-conservative tests: Terms usually encountered in discussions of *multiple comparison tests*. Non-conservative tests provide poor control over the *per-experiment error rate*. Conservative tests, on the other hand, may limit the *per-comparison error rate* to unnecessarily low values, and tend to have low *power* unless the sample size is large.

Consistency: A term used for a particular property of an estimator, namely, that its *bias* tends to zero as sample size increases.

Consistency checks: Checks built into the collection of a set of observations to assess their internal consistency. For example, data on age might be collected directly and also by asking about date of birth.

Consultation times: Several authors have shown that the distribution of consultation times at doctors' surgeries can be satisfactorily fitted by a *gamma distribution*, and that the mean consultation time is in the range 2–10 minutes.

Contact rate: See **Rvachev–Baroyan–Longini model**.

Contagious distribution: A term used for the *probability distribution* of the sum of a number (N) of *random variables*, particularly when N is also a random variable. For example, if $x_1, x_2, \cdots, x_N$ are variables with a *Bernoulli distribution* and N is a variable having a *Poisson distribution* with mean λ, then the sum S_N, given by

$$S_N = x_1 + x_2 + \cdots + x_N$$

can be shown to have a Poisson distribution with mean λp, where $p = \mathrm{P}(x_i = 1)$. See also **compound distribution**.

Contaminated normal distribution: A term sometimes used for a *finite mixture distribution* of two *normal distributions* with the same mean but different variances. Such distributions have often been used in applications of *Monte Carlo methods*.

Content analysis: The coding of statements or answers to open-ended questions made in relatively unstructured interviews.

Contingency coefficient: A measure of association, C, of the two variables forming a *two-dimensional contingency table*, given by

$$C = \sqrt{\frac{X^2}{X^2 + N}}$$

where X^2 is the usual *chi-squared statistic* for testing the independence of the two variables and N is the sample size. See also **phi-coefficient**.

Contingency tables: The tables arising when observations on a number of *categorical variables* are cross-classified. Entries in each cell are the number of individuals with the corresponding combination of variable values. Most common are tables involving two categorical variables known as *two-dimensional contingency tables*, an example of which is shown below;

Retarded activity amongst psychiatric patients

	Affectives	Schizo	Neurotics	Total
Retarded activity	12	13	5	30
No retarded activity	18	17	25	60
Total	30	30	30	90

The analysis of such two-dimensional tables generally involves testing for the independence of the two variables using the familiar *chi-squared statistic*. Three- and higher-dimensional tables are now routinely analysed using *log-linear models*.

Continual reassessment method: An approach that applies *Bayesian inference* to determining the *maximum tolerated dose* in a *phase I trial*. The method begins by assuming a *logistic regression* model for the dose-toxicity relationship and a *prior distribution* for the parameters. After each patient's toxicity result becomes available, the *posterior distribution* of the parameters is recomputed and used to estimate the probability of toxicity at each of a series of dose levels.

Continuity correction: See **Yates' correction**.

Continuous screen design: See **screening studies**.

Continuous variable: A measurement not restricted to particular values except in so far as this is restricted by the accuracy of the measuring instrument. Common examples include weight, height, temperature, and blood pressure. For such a variable, equal sized differences on different parts of the scale are equivalent. See also **categorical variable** and **ordinal variable**.

Contour plot: A topographical map drawn from data involving observations on three variables. One variable is represented on the horizontal axis and a second variable is represented on the vertical axis. The third variable is represented by isolines (lines of constant value). These plots are often helpful in data analysis, especially when searching for maxima or minima in such data. The plots are most often used to display graphically *bivariate distributions*, in which case the third variable is the value of the *prob-*

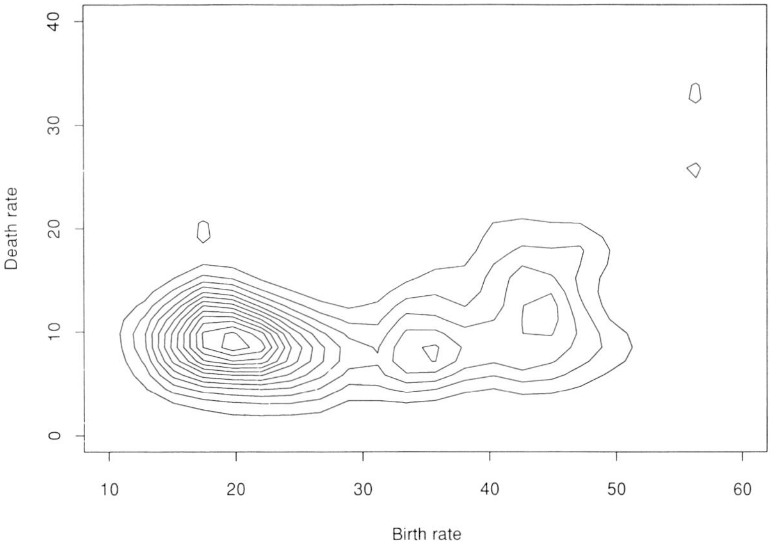

Fig 16 Contour plot of bivariate distribution of birth and death rates.

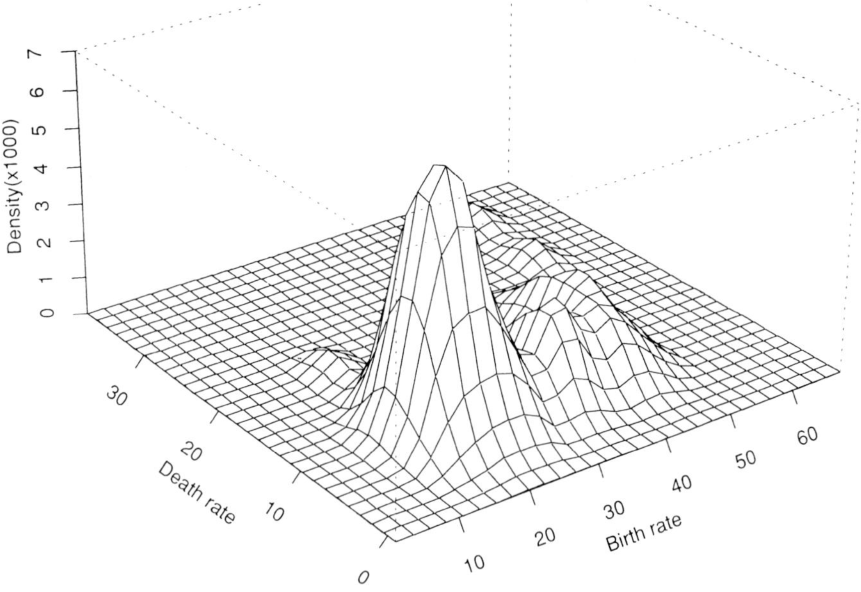

Fig 17 Perspective plot of bivariate distribution of birth and death rates.

ability density function corresponding to the values of the two variables. An alternative method of displaying the same material is provided by the *perspective plot*, in which the values of the third variable are represented by a series of lines constructed to give a three-dimensional view of the data.

Contrast: A *linear function* of parameters or statistics in which the coefficients sum to zero. Most often encountered in the context of *analysis of variance*. For example, in an application involving, say, three treatment groups (with means $\bar{x}_{T_1}$, $\bar{x}_{T_2}$ and $\bar{x}_{T_3}$) and a control group (with mean $\bar{x}_C$), the following is the contrast for comparing the mean of the control group with the average of the treatment groups:

$$\bar{x}_C - \tfrac{1}{3}\bar{x}_{T_1} - \tfrac{1}{3}\bar{x}_{T_2} - \tfrac{1}{3}\bar{x}_{T_3}$$

See also **Helmert contrast** and **orthogonal contrast**.

Control chart: See **quality control procedures**.

Control group: In *experimental studies*, a collection of individuals to which the experimental procedure of interest is not applied. In *observational studies*, most often used for a collection of individuals not subjected to the *risk factor* under investigation. In many studies, the controls are drawn from the same clinical source as the cases, to ensure that they represent the same catchment population and are subject to the same selective factors. These would be termed *hospital controls*. An alternative is to use controls taken from the population from which the cases are drawn (*community controls*). The latter is suitable only if the source population is well defined and the cases are representative of the cases in this population.

Controlled trial: A *phase III clinical trial* in which an experimental treatment is compared with a control treatment, the latter being either the current standard treatment or a placebo.

Control statistics: Statistics calculated from sample values $x_1, x_2, \cdots, x_n$ which elicit information about some characteristic of a process which is being monitored. The sample mean, for example, is often used to monitor the mean level of a process, and the sample variance its imprecision. See also **cusum** and **quality control procedures**.

Convex hull: See **convex hull trimming**.

Convex hull trimming: A procedure that can be applied to a set of *bivariate data* to allow *robust estimation* of *Pearson's product moment correlation coefficient*. The points defining the *convex hull* of the observations, i.e., the vertices of the smallest convex polyhedron in variable space within or on which all the data points lie, are deleted before the correlation coefficient is calculated. The major attraction of this method is that it eliminates isolated *outliers* without disturbing the general shape of the bivariate distribution.

Convolution: An integral (or sum) used to obtain the *probability distribution* of the sum of two or more *random variables*.

Cook's distance: A measure of the change that would occur in the estimated parameters in some model of interest if a particular observation was omitted. Useful in identifying observations that have the greatest *influence* on the estimation of parameters.

Cooperative study: A term sometimes used for *multicentre study*.

Cophenetic correlation: The correlation between the observed values in a *similarity matrix* or *dissimilarity matrix* and the corresponding fusion levels in the *dendrogram* obtained by applying an *agglomerative hierarchical clustering method* to the matrix. Used as a measure of how well the clustering matches the data.

Coplot: A powerful visualization tool for studying how a response depends on an explanatory variable, given the values of other explanatory variables. The plot consists of a number of panels, one of which (the 'given' panel) shows the values of a particular explanatory variable divided into a number of intervals, whilst the others (the 'dependence' panels) show the *scatterplots* of the response variable and another explanatory variable corresponding to each interval in the given panel. The plot is examined by moving from left to right through the intervals in the given panel, while simultaneously moving from left to right and then from bottom to top through the dependence panels. The example shown involves the relationship between packed cell volume and white blood cell count for given haemoglobin concentration.

Correlated binary data: Synonym for **clustered binary data**.

Correlated samples t-test: Synonym for **matched pairs t-test**.

Correlation: A general term for interdependence between pairs of variables. See also **association**.

Correlation coefficient: An index that quantifies the linear relationship between a pair of variables. In a *bivariate normal distribution*, for example, the parameter ρ. For sample observations, a variety of such coefficients have been suggested, of which the most commonly used is *Pearson's product moment correlation coefficient*, defined as

$$r = \frac{\sum_{i=1}^{n}(x_i - \bar{x})(y_i - \bar{y})}{\sqrt{\sum_{i=1}^{n}(x_i - \bar{x})^2(y_i - \bar{y})^2}}$$

where $(x_1, y_1), (x_2, y_2), \cdots, (x_n, y_n)$ are the n sample values of the two

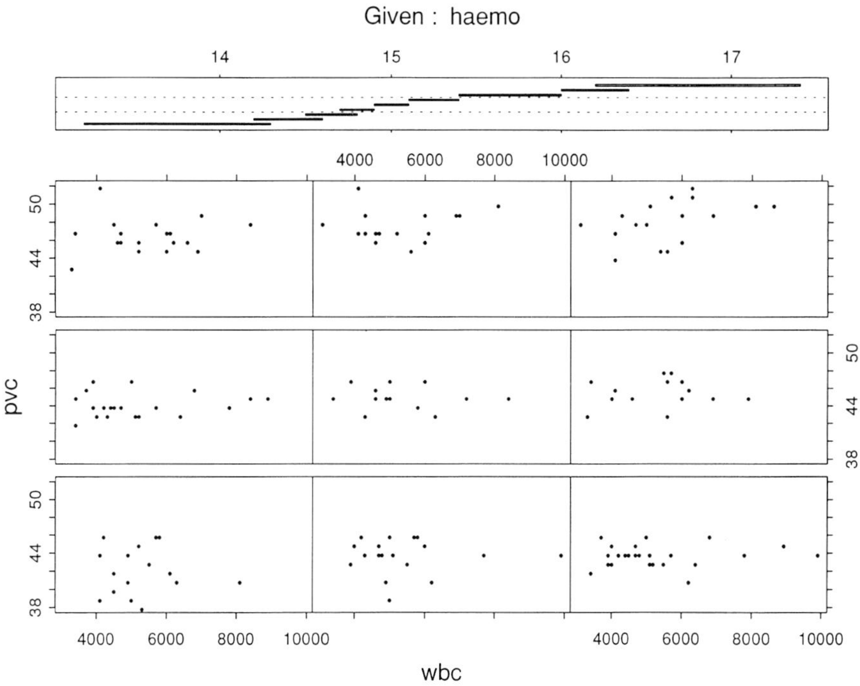

Fig 18 Coplot of haemoglobin concentration, packed cell volume and white blood cell count.

variables of interest. The coefficient takes values between -1 and 1, with the sign indicating the direction of the relationship and the numerical magnitude its strength. Values of -1 or 1 indicate that the sample values fall on a straight line. A value of zero indicates the lack of any linear relationship between the two variables. See also **Spearman's rho, intraclass correlation** and **Kendall's tau statistics**.

Correlation matrix: A square, *symmetric matrix* with rows and columns corresponding to variables, in which the off-diagonal elements are correlations between pairs of variables, and elements on the main diagonal are unity. An example for measures of muscle and body fat is as follows,:

Correlation matrix for muscle, skin and body fat data

$$\mathbf{R} = \begin{array}{c} \\ V1 \\ V2 \\ V3 \\ V4 \end{array} \begin{array}{c} \begin{array}{cccc} V1 & V2 & V3 & V4 \end{array} \\ \begin{pmatrix} 1.00 & 0.92 & 0.46 & 0.84 \\ 0.92 & 1.00 & 0.08 & 0.88 \\ 0.46 & 0.08 & 1.00 & 0.14 \\ 0.84 & 0.88 & 0.14 & 1.00 \end{pmatrix} \end{array}$$

V1 = Tricep (thickness, mm), V2 = Thigh (circumference, mm), V3 = Midarm (circumference, mm), V4 = Bodyfat (%).

Correlogram: See **autocorrelation**.

Correspondence analysis: A method for deriving a set of coordinate values representing the row and column categories of a *contingency table*, and thus allowing the associations in the table to be displayed graphically. The derived coordinates are analogous to those resulting from a *principal components analysis*, except that they involve a partition of a *chi-squared statistic* rather than the total variance. The example shown arises from the following table:

Eye Colour			**Hair Colour**		
	Fair	Red	Medium	Dark	Black
Light	688	116	584	188	4
Blue	326	38	241	110	3
Medium	343	84	909	412	26
Dark	98	48	403	681	81

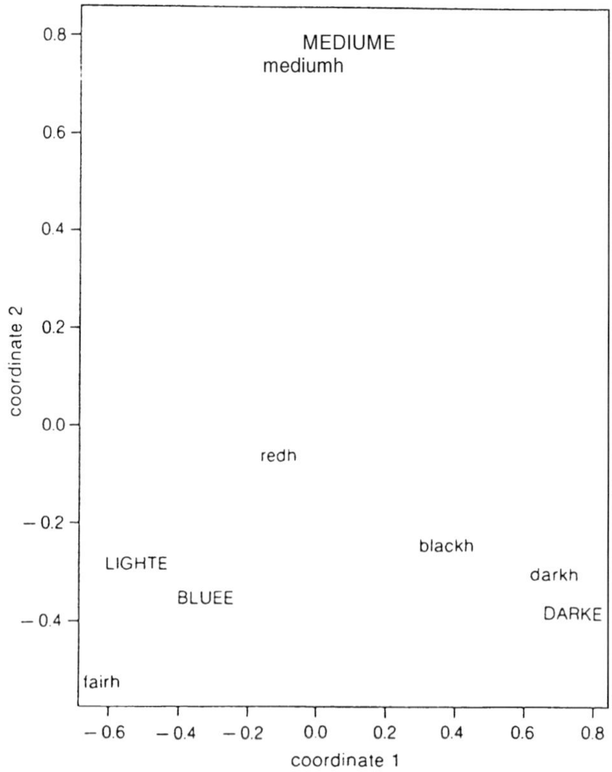

Fig 19 Correspondence analysis plot derived from hair colour/eye colour data.

Cosinor analysis: The analysis of biological rhythm data, that is, data with *circadian variation*, generally by fitting a single sinusoidal regression function having a known period of 24 hours, together with independent and identically distributed error terms.

Cost–benefit analysis: An economic analysis in which the costs of medical care and the loss of net earnings due to death or disability are considered.

Count data: Data obtained by counting the number of occurrences of particular events, rather than by taking measurements on some scale.

Covariance: The *expected value* of the product of the deviations of two *random variables*, x and y, from their respective means, μ_x and μ_y, i.e.,

$$\text{Cov}(x, y) = E(x - \mu_x)(y - \mu_y)$$

The corresponding sample statistic is

$$c_{xy} = \frac{1}{n}\sum_{i=1}^{n}(x_i - \bar{x})(y_i - \bar{y})$$

where (x_i, y_i), $i = 1, \cdots, n$ are the sample values on the two variables, and $\bar{x}$ and $\bar{y}$ their respective means. See also **variance–covariance matrix** and **correlation coefficient**.

Covariance matrix: See **variance–covariance matrix**.

Covariance structure models: Synonym for **structural equation models**.

Covariates: Often used simply as an alternative name for explanatory variables, but perhaps more specifically to refer to variables that are not of primary interest in an investigation, but are measured because it is believed that they are likely to affect the response variable, and consequently need to be included in analyses and model building.

Cox–Mantel test: A *distribution-free method* for comparing two *survival curves*. Assuming $t_{(1)}, < t_{(2)}, < \cdots, < t_{(k)}$ to be the distinct *survival times* in the two groups, the *test statistic* is

$$C = U/\sqrt{I}$$

where

$$U = r_2 - \sum_{i=1}^{k} m_{(i)} A_{(i)}$$

$$I = \sum_{i=1}^{k} \frac{m_{(i)}(r_{(i)} - m_{(i)})}{r_{(i)} - 1} A_{(i)}(1 - A_{(i)})$$

In these formulae, r_2 is the number of individuals in the second group,

$r_{(i)}$ the total number of individuals who died or were censored at time $t_{(i)}$, $m_{(i)}$ the number of survival times equal to $t_{(i)}$, and $A_{(i)}$ is the proportion of these individuals in group two. If the survival experience of the two groups is the same then C has a *standard normal distribution.*

Cox–Snell residuals: Residuals widely used in the analysis of *survival time* data and defined as

$$r_i = -\ln \hat{S}_i(t_i)$$

where $\hat{S}_i(t_i)$ is the estimated *survival function* of the i-th individual at the observed *survival time* of t_i. If the correct model has been fitted, then these residuals will be n observations from an *exponential distribution* with mean unity.

Cox's proportional hazards model: A method that allows the *hazard function* to be modelled on a set of explanatory variables without making restrictive assumptions about the dependence of the hazard function on time. The model involved is

$$\ln h(t) = \ln \alpha(t) + \beta_1 x_1 + \beta_2 x_2 + \cdots + \beta_q x_q$$

where $x_1, x_2, \cdots, x_q$ are the explanatory variables of interest, and $h(t)$ the hazard function. The so-called *baseline hazard function*, $\alpha(t)$, is an arbitrary function of time. For any two individuals at any point in time, the ratio of the hazard functions is a constant. Because the baseline hazard function, $\alpha(t)$, does not have to specified explicitly, the procedure is essentially a *distribution-free method.* Estimates of the parameters in the model, i.e., $\beta_1, \beta_2, \cdots, \beta_p$, are usually obtained by *maximum likelihood estimation*, and depend only on the order in which events occur, not on the exact times of their occurrence.

Cramer's V: A measure of association for the two variables forming a *two-dimensional contingency table.* Related to the *phi-coefficient*, ϕ, but applicable to tables larger than 2×2. The coefficient is given by

$$V = \sqrt{\left\{\frac{\phi^2}{\min[(r-1)(c-1)]}\right\}}$$

where r is the number of rows of the table and c is the number of columns. See also **contingency coefficient**.

Cramer–von Mises test: A test of whether a set of observations arise from a *normal distribution.* The *test statistic* is

$$W = \sum_{i=1}^{n}\left[z_i - \frac{(2i-1)^2}{2n}\right] + \frac{1}{12n}$$

where the z_i are found from the ordered sample values,

$x_{(1)} \le x_{(2)} \le \cdots \le x_{(n)}$, as

$$z_i = \int_{-\infty}^{x_{(i)}} \frac{1}{\sqrt{2\pi}} e^{-\frac{1}{2}u^2} du.$$

Critical values of W can be found in many sets of statistical tables.

Critical region: The values of a *test statistic* that lead to rejection of a *null hypothesis*. The size of the critical region is the probability of obtaining an outcome belonging to this region when the null hypothesis is true, i.e., the probability of a *type I error*. See also **acceptance region**.

Critical value: The value with which a statistic calculated from sample data is compared in order to decide whether a *null hypothesis* should be rejected. The value is related to the particular significance level chosen.

Cronbach's alpha: An index of the internal consistency of a psychological test. If the test consists of n items and an individual's score is the total answered correctly, then the coefficient is given specifically by

$$\alpha = \frac{n}{n-1}\left[1 - \frac{1}{\sigma^2}\sum_{i=1}^{n}\sigma_i^2\right]$$

where σ^2 is the variance of the total scores and σ_i^2 is the variance of the set of 0,1 scores representing correct and incorrect answers on item i.

Cross-correlation function: The correlations between the values of two *time series*, x_t, y_t, for a range of values of the lag between them.

Cross-cultural study: A study in which data from different cultural groups are compared.

Crossed treatments: Two or more treatments that are used in sequence (as in a *crossover design*) or in combination (as in a *factorial design*).

Crossover design: A type of *longitudinal study* in which subjects receive different treatments on different occasions. *Random allocation* is used to determine the order in which the treatments are received. The simplest such design involves two groups of subjects, one of which receives each of two treatments, A and B, in the order AB, while the other receives them in the reverse order. This is known as a *two-by-two crossover design*. Since the treatment comparison is 'within subject' rather than 'between subject', it is likely to require fewer subjects to achieve a given *power*. The analysis of such designs is not necessarily straightforward because of the possibility of *carryover effects*, that is, residual effects of the treatment received on the first occasion that remain present into the second occasion. An attempt to minimize this problem is often made by including a *wash-out period* between the two treatment occasions. Some authorities have suggested that this type of design should only be used if such carry-over effects can be ruled out *a priori*. Crossover designs are only applicable to chronic conditions for which short-term relief of symptoms is the goal rather than a cure. See also **three-period crossover designs**.

Crossover rate: The proportion of patients in a *clinical trial* transferring from the treatment decided by an initial *random allocation* to an alternative one.

Cross-sectional study: A study not involving the passing of time. All information is collected at the same time and subjects are contacted only once. Many surveys are of this type. The temporal sequence of cause and effect cannot be addressed in such a study, but it may be suggestive of an association that should be investigated more fully by, for example, a *prospective study*.

Cross-validation: The division of data into two approximately equal sized subsets, one of which is used to estimate the parameters in some model of interest, and the other is used to assess whether the model with these parameter values fits adequately. See also **jackknife**.

Crowding index: The mean number of persons per room in a housing unit.

Crude death rate: The total deaths during a year divided by the total midyear population. To avoid many decimal places, it is customary to multiply death rates by 100 000 and express the results as deaths per 100 000 population. See also **age-specific death rates** and **cause-specific death rates**.

Cubic spline: See **spline functions**.

Cumulative distribution function: A distribution showing how many values of a *random variable* are less than or more than given values. For grouped data the given values correspond to the class boundaries.

Cumulative frequency distribution: A listing of the sample values of a variable, together with the proportion of the observations less than or equal to each value. See also **frequency distribution**.

Cumulative hazard function: A function, $H(t)$, used in the analysis of data involving *survival times* and given by

$$H(t) = \int_0^t h(u)\mathrm{d}u$$

where $h(t)$ is the *hazard function*. Can also be written in terms of the *survival function*, $S(t)$, as $H(t) = -\ln S(t)$.

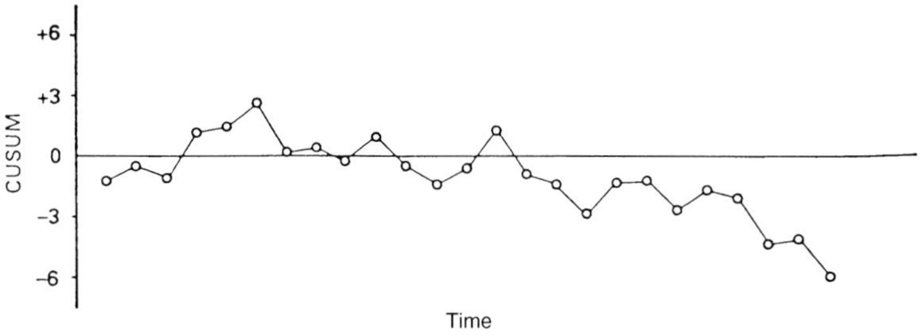

Fig 20 Cusum chart.

Cusum: A procedure for investigating the influence of time even when it is not part of the design of a study. For a series $X_1, X_2, \cdots, X_n$, the cusum series is defined as

$$S_i = \sum_{j=1}^{i} (X_j - X_0)$$

where X_0 is a reference level representing an initial or normal value for the data. Depending on the application, X_0 may be chosen to be the mean of the series, the mean of the first few observations or some value justified by theory. If the true mean is X_0 and there is no time trend then the cusum is basically flat. A change in level of the raw data over time appears as a change in the slope of the cusum.

Cuzick's trend test: A *distribution-free method* for testing the trend in a measured variable across a series of ordered groups. The *test statistic* for a sample of N subjects is given by

$$T = \sum_{i=1}^{N} Z_i r_i$$

where $Z_i (i = 1, \cdots, N)$ is the group index for subject i (this may be one of the numbers $1, \cdots, G$ arranged in some natural order, where G is the number of groups, or, for example, a measure of exposure for the group), and r_i is the rank of the ith subject's observation in the combined sample. Under the *null hypothesis* that there is no trend across groups, the mean (μ) and variance (σ^2) of T are given by

$$\mu = N(N+1)E(Z)/2$$
$$\sigma^2 = N^2(N+1)V(Z)/12$$

where $E(Z)$ and $V(Z)$ are the calculated mean and variance of the Z_i values.

Cycle: A term used when referring to *time series* for a periodic movement of the series. The *period* of the series is the time it takes for one complete up-and-down and down-and-up movement.

Cycle plot: A graphical method for studying the behaviour of seasonal *time series*. In such a plot, the January values of the seasonal component are graphed for successive years, then the February values are graphed, and so forth. For each monthly subseries the mean of the values is represented by a horizontal line. The graph allows an assessment of the overall pattern of the seasonal change, as portrayed by the horizontal mean lines, as well as the behaviour of each monthly subseries. Since all of the latter are on the same graph it is readily seen whether the change in any subseries is large or small compared with that in the overall pattern of the seasonal component.

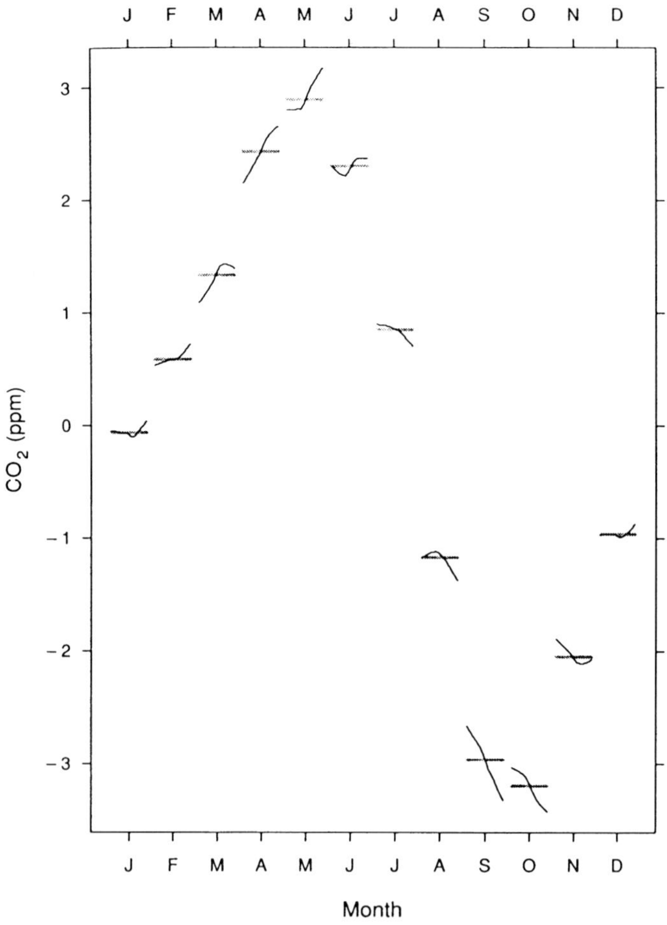

Fig 21 Cycle plot of carbon dioxide concentrations.

Cyclic variation: The systematic and repeatable variation of some variable over time. Most people's blood pressure, for example, shows such variation over a 24 hour period, being lowest at night and highest during the morning. Such *circadian variation* is also seen in many hormone levels.

D

D'Agostino's test: A test based on ordered sample values, $x_{(1)} \leq x_{(2)} \leq \cdots \leq x_{(n)}$, with mean $\bar{x}$, used to assess whether the observations arise from a *normal distribution*. The *test statistic* is

$$D = \frac{\sum_{i=1}^{n}\{i - \frac{1}{2}(n+1)\}x_{(i)}}{n\sqrt{n\sum_{i=1}^{n}(x_{(i)} - \bar{x})^2}}$$

Appropriate for testing depatures from normality due either to *skewness* or to the distribution not being *mesokurtoic*. Tables of *critical values* are available.

Darling test: A test that a set of *random variables* arises from an *exponential distribution*. If $x_1, x_2, \cdots, x_n$ are the n sample values, the *test statistic* is

$$K_m = \frac{\sum_{i=1}^{n}(x_i - \bar{x})^2}{\bar{x}^2}$$

where $\bar{x}$ is the mean of the sample. Asymptotically K_m can be shown to have mean (μ) and variance (σ^2) given by

$$\mu = \frac{n(n-1)}{n+1}$$

$$\sigma^2 = \frac{4n^4(n-1)}{(n+1)^2(n+2)(n+3)}$$

so that $z = \frac{(K_m - \mu)}{\sigma}$ has asymptotically a *standard normal distribution* under the exponential distribution hypothesis.

Data augmentation: A scheme for augmenting observed data so as to make it more easy to analyse. A simple example is the estimation of *missing values* to balance a *factorial design* with different numbers of observations in each cell. The term is most often used in respect of an iterative procedure common in the computation of the *posterior distribution* in *Bayesian inference*. See also **Gibbs sampling**.

Database: A structured collection of data that is organised in such a way that it may be accessed easily by a wide variety of applications programs. Large clinical databases are becoming increasingly available to clinical and policy researchers; they are generally used for two purposes: to facilitate health care delivery, and for research. An example of such a database is that provided by the US Health Care Financing Administration, which contains information about all Medicare patients' hospitalizations, surgical procedures and office visits.

Database management system: A computer system organised for the systematic management of a large structured collection of information, that can be used for storage, modification and retrieval of data.

Data dredging: A term used to describe comparisons made within a data set not specifically prescribed prior to the start of the study. See also **subgroup analysis**.

Data editing: The action of removing format errors and keying errors from data.

Data matrix: See **multivariate data**.

Data reduction: The process of summarizing large amounts of data by forming *frequency distributions*, *histograms*, *scatter diagrams*, etc., and calculating statistics such as means, variances and correlation coefficients. The term is also used when obtaining a low-dimensional representation of *multivariate data* by procedures such as *principal components* and *factor analysis*.

Data set: A general term for observations and measurements collected during any type of scientific investigation.

Data screening: The initial assessment of a set of observations to see whether or not they appear to satisfy the assumptions of the methods to be used in their analysis. Techniques which highlight possible *outliers*, or, for example, departures from normality, such as a *normal probability plot*, are important in this phase of an investigation. See also **initial data analysis**.

Data smoothing algorithms: Procedures for extracting a pattern in a sequence of observations when this is obscured by *noise*. Basically, any such technique separates the original series into a smooth sequence and a residual sequence (commonly called the 'rough'). For example, a smoother can separate seasonal fluctuations from briefer events such as identifiable peaks and random noise. A simple example of such a procedure is the *moving average*; a more complex one is the *lowess* smoother. See also **Kalman filter**.

Death rate: See **crude death rate**.

Debugging: The process of locating and correcting errors in a computer routine, or of isolating and eliminating malfunctions of a computer itself.

Deciles: The values of a variable that divide its *probability distribution* or its *frequency distribution* into ten equal parts.

Decimal reduction time: A parameter used to measure the efficacy of the thermal disinfection of microbial populations, given by the time required to reduce the population by 90% .

Decision function: See **decision theory**.

Decision theory: A unified approach to all problems of estimation, prediction, and hypothesis testing. It is based on the concept of a *decision function*, which tells the experimenter how to conduct the statistical aspects of an experiment and what action to take for each possible outcome. Choosing a decision function requires a *loss function* to be defined which assigns numerical values to making good or poor decisions.

Decision tree: A graphic representation of the alternatives in a decision making problem that summarizes all the possibilities foreseen by the decision maker. For example, suppose we are given the following problem:

A physician must choose between two treatments. The patient is known to have one of two diseases but the diagnosis is not certain. A

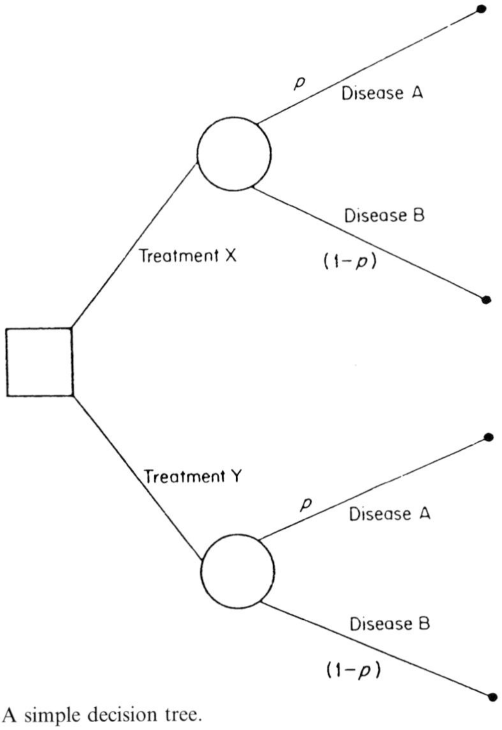

Fig 22 A simple decision tree.

through examination of the patient was not able to resolve the diagnostic uncertainty. The best that can be said is that the probability that the patient has disease A is p. A simple decision tree for the problem is given.

Deep models: A term used for those models applied in *screening studies* that incorporate hypotheses about the disease process that generates the observed events. The aim of such models is to attempt an understanding of the underlying disease dynamics. See also **surface models**.

Degrees of freedom (df): An elusive concept that occurs throughout statistics. Essentially, the term means the number of independent units of information in a sample relevant to the estimation of a parameter or calculation of a statistic. For example, in a *two-by-two contingency table* with a given set of marginal totals, only one of the four cell frequencies is free, and the table has therefore a single degree of freedom. In many cases the term corresponds to the number of parameters in a model. Also used to refer to a parameter of various families of distributions, for example, *Student's t-distribution* and the *F-distribution*.

Delta(δ) technique: A procedure that uses the *Taylor series expansion* of a function of one or more *random variables* to obtain approximations to the *expected value* of the function and to its variance.

Demography: The study of human populations by statistical methods.

DeMoivre–Laplace theorem: This theorem states that, if x is a *random variable* having the *binomial distribution* with parameters n and p, then the *asymptotic distribution* of x is a *normal distribution* with mean np and variance $np(1-p)$. See also **normal approximation**.

Dendrogram: A term usually encountered in the application of *agglomerative hierarchical clustering methods*, where it refers to the 'tree-like' diagram illustrating the series of steps taken by the method in proceeding from n single member 'clusters' to a single group containing all n individuals. The example shown in fig. 23 arises from applying *single linkage clustering* to the following matrix of *Euclidean distances* between five points:

$$\mathbf{D} = \begin{pmatrix} 0.0 & & & & \\ 2.0 & 0.0 & & & \\ 6.0 & 5.0 & 0.0 & & \\ 10.0 & 9.0 & 4.0 & 0.0 & \\ 9.0 & 8.0 & 5.0 & 3.0 & 0.0 \end{pmatrix}$$

Density estimation: Procedures for estimating *probability distributions* without assuming any particular functional form. Constructing a *histogram* is

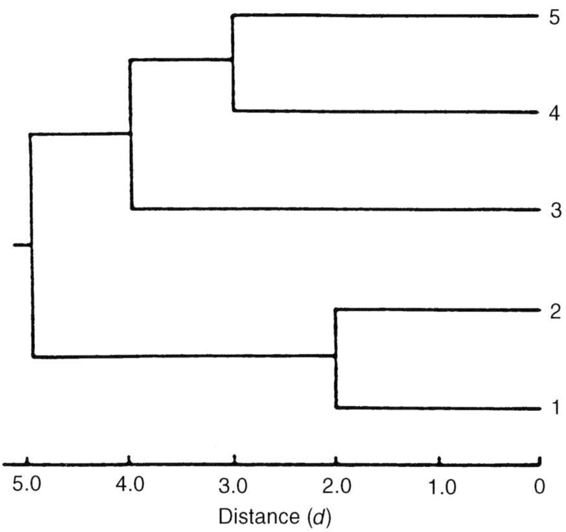

Fig 23 A dendrogram.

perhaps the simplest example of such estimation, and *kernel methods* illustrate a more sophisticated approach.

Density function: See **probability density**.

Dependent variable: See **response variable**.

Descriptive statistics: A general term for methods of summarizing and tabulating data that make their main features more transparent; for example, calculating means and variances and plotting histograms. See also **exploratory data analysis** and **initial data analysis**.

Design matrix: A matrix that specifies a statistical model for a set of observations. For example, in a *one-way design* with three observations in one group, two observations in a second group and a single observation in the third group, and where the model is

$$y_{ij} = \mu + \alpha_i + \epsilon_{ij}$$

the design matrix, **X** is

$$\mathbf{X} = \begin{pmatrix} 1 & 1 & 0 & 0 \\ 1 & 1 & 0 & 0 \\ 1 & 1 & 0 & 0 \\ 1 & 0 & 1 & 0 \\ 1 & 0 & 1 & 0 \\ 1 & 0 & 0 & 1 \end{pmatrix}$$

Using this matrix, the model for all the observations can be conveniently expressed in matrix form as

$$\mathbf{y} = \mathbf{X}\boldsymbol{\beta} + \boldsymbol{\epsilon}$$

where $\mathbf{y}' = [y_{11}, y_{12}, y_{13}, y_{21}, y_{22}, y_{31}]$, $\boldsymbol{\beta}' = [\mu, \alpha_1, \alpha_2, \alpha_3]$ and $\boldsymbol{\epsilon}' = [\epsilon_{11}, \epsilon_{12}, \epsilon_{13}, \epsilon_{21}, \epsilon_{22}, \epsilon_{31}]$.

Design set: Synonym for **training set**.

Detectable preclinical period: Synonym for **sojourn time**.

Detection bias: See **ascertainment bias**.

Determinant: A value associated with a *square matrix* that represents sums and products of its elements. For example, if the matrix is

$$\mathbf{A} = \begin{pmatrix} a & b \\ c & d \end{pmatrix}$$

then the determinant of **A** (conventionally written as det(**A**) or $|\mathbf{A}|$) is given by

$$ad - bc$$

Deterministic model: One that contains no random or probabilistic elements. See also **random model**.

Detrending: A term used in the analysis of *time series* data for the process of calculating a *trend* in some way and then subtracting the trend values from those of the original series.

Deviance: A measure of the extent to which a particular model differs from the *saturated model* for a data set. Defined explicitly in terms of the *likelihoods* of the two models as

$$D = -2[\ln L_c - \ln L_s]$$

where L_c and L_s are the likelihoods of the current model and the saturated model, respectively. Large values of D are encountered when L_c is small relative to L_s, indicating that the current model is a poor one. Small values of D are obtained in the reverse case. The deviance has, asymptotically, a *chi-squared distribution* with degrees of freedom equal to the difference in the number of parameters in the two models. See also **$\mathbf{G}^2$** and **likelihood ratio**.

Deviate: The value of a variable measured from some standard point of location, usually the mean.

DF(df): Abbreviation for **degrees of freedom**.

Diagnostic tests: Procedures used in clinical medicine and also in *epidemiology*, to screen for the presence or absence of a disease. In the simplest case, the test will result in a positive (disease likely) or negative (disease unlikely) finding. Ideally, all those with the disease should be classified by the test as positive and all those without the disease as negative. Two indices of the performance of a test which measure how often such correct classifications occur are its *sensitivity* and *specificity*. See also **Bayes' theorem** and **believe the positive rule**.

Diagonal matrix: A *square matrix* whose off-diagonal elements are all zero. For example:

$$\mathbf{D} = \begin{pmatrix} 10 & 0 & 0 \\ 0 & 5 & 0 \\ 0 & 0 & 3 \end{pmatrix}$$

Dichotomous variable: Synonym for **binary variable**.

Dietz, Molineaux and Thomas model: A mathematical model for the transmission of malaria.

Differences vs totals plot: A graphical procedure most often used in the analysis of data from a *two-by-two crossover design*. For each subject, the difference between the response variable values on each treatment are plotted against the total of the two treatment values. The two groups, corresponding to the order in which the treatments were given, are differentiated on the plot by different plotting symbols (in the example given, Fig. 24, 'AB' and 'BA' are used). A large shift between the groups in the horizontal direction implies a differential *carryover effect*. If this shift is small, then the shift between the groups in a vertical direction is a measure of the treatment effect.

Differencing: A simple approach to removing *trends* in *time series*. The first difference of a time series, $\{y_t\}$ is defined as the transformation

$$\mathrm{D}y_t = y_t - y_{t-1}$$

Higher-order differences are defined by repeated application. So, for example, the second difference, $\mathrm{D}^2 y_t$, is given by

$$\mathrm{D}^2 y_t = \mathrm{D}(\mathrm{D}y_t) = \mathrm{D}y_t - \mathrm{D}y_{t-1} = y_t - 2y_{t-1} + y_{t-2}$$

Frequently used in practice to achieve a *stationary series* before fitting models. See also **backward shift operator** and **autoregressive integrated moving average models**.

Digit preference: The personal and often subconscious bias that frequently occurs in the recording of observations. Usually most obvious in the final recorded digit of a measurement.

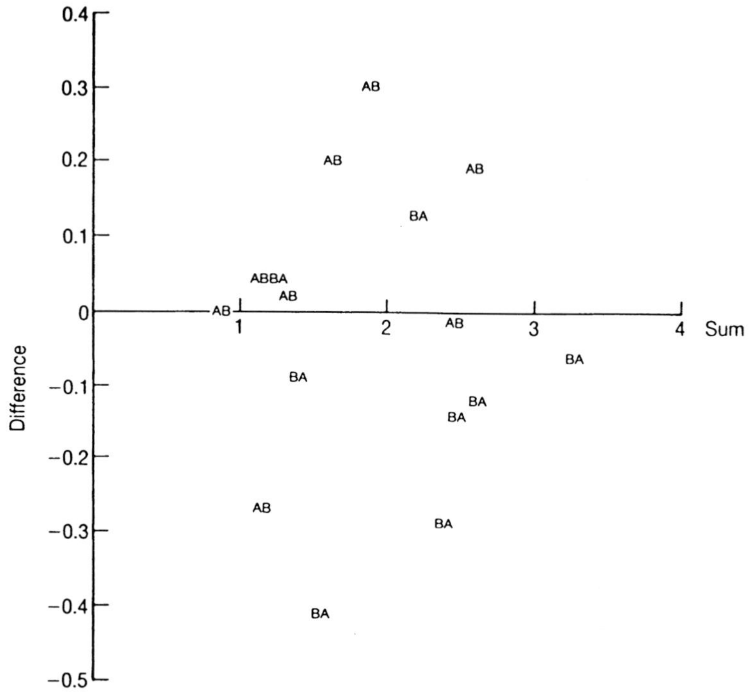

Fig 24 Differences versus totals plot.

Digraph: Synonym for **directed graph**.

DIP test: A test for whether a population has a *unimodal distribution* or a *multimodal distribution*.

Directed graph: See **graph theory**.

Direct matrix product: Synonym for **Kronecker product**.

Direct standardization: The process of adjusting a crude mortality or morbidity rate estimate for one or more variables, by using a known *reference population*. It might, for example, be required to compare cancer mortality rates of single and married women with adjustment being made for the age distribution of the two groups, which is very likely to differ with the married women being older. *Age-specific death rates* derived from each of the two groups would be applied to the population age distribution, to yield mortality rates that could be directly compared. See also **indirect standardization**.

Dirichlet distribution: A *multivariate distribution* that is the multivariate version of the *beta distribution*. Given by

$$f(x_1, x_2, \cdots, x_q) = \frac{\Gamma(\nu_1 + \cdots + \nu_{q+1})}{\Gamma(\nu_1)\cdots\Gamma(\nu_{q+1})} x_1^{\nu_1 - 1} \cdots x_q^{\nu_q - 1}$$
$$\times (1 - x_1 - \cdots - x_q)^{\nu_{q+1} - 1}$$

where the *random variables* $x_1, x_2, \cdots, x_q$ are such that $x_i \geq 0, i = 1, \cdots, q$, and $\sum x_i \leq 1$.

Dirichlet tessellation: A construction for events that occur in some planar region A, consisting of a series of 'territories', each of which consists of that part of A closer to a particular event x_i than to any other event x_j.

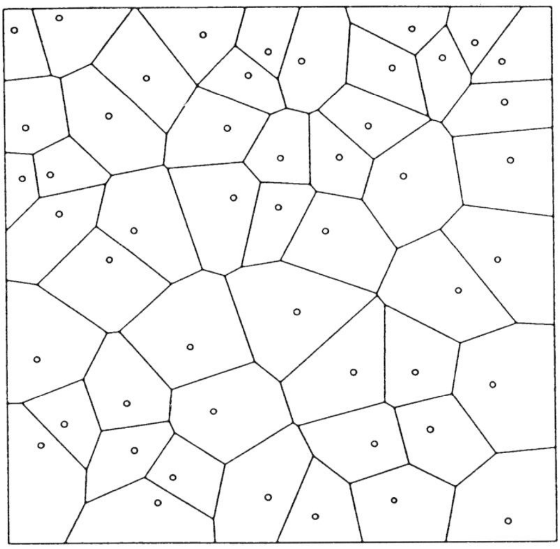

Fig 25 An example of a Dirichlet tesselation.

Discontinuation rate: A term specific to studies of contraceptives, given by the total number of discontinuations of a device divided by the number of people continuing to use the device.

Discrete variables: Variables having only integer values, for example, number of births, number of pregnancies, number of teeth extracted.

Discriminant analysis: A term that covers a large number of techniques for the analysis of *multivariate data*, that have in common the aim to assess whether or not a set of variables distinguish or discriminate between two (or more) groups of individuals. In medicine, such methods are generally applied to the problem of using optimally the results from a number of tests, or the observations of a number of symptoms, to make a diagnosis that can only be confirmed perhaps by post-mortem examination. In the two group case the most commonly used method is *Fisher's linear discriminant function*, in which a *linear function* of the variables giving maximal separation between the groups is determined. This results in a *classification rule* (often also known as an *allocation rule*) that may be used to assign a new patient to one of the two groups. The derivation of this linear function assumes that the *variance–covariance matrices* of the two groups are the same. If they are not then a *quadratic discriminant function* may be necessary to distinguish between the groups. Such a function contains powers and cross-products of variables. The sample of observations from which the discriminant function is derived is often known as the *training set*. When more than two groups are involved (all with the same variance–covariance matrix), then it is possible to determine several linear functions of the variables for separating them. In general, the number of such functions that can be derived is the smaller of q and $g - 1$, where q is the number of variables and g the number of groups. The collection of linear functions for discrimination are known as *canonical discriminant functions* or often simply as *canonical variates*.

Disease cluster: An unusual aggregation of health events, real or perceived. The events may be grouped in a particular area or in some short period of time, or they may occur among a certain group of people, for example, those having a particular occupation. The significance of studying such clusters as a means of determining the origins of public health problems has long been recognized. In 1850, for example, the Broad Street pump in London was identified as a major source of cholera by plotting cases on a map and noting the cluster around the well. More recently, recognition of clusters of relatively rare kinds of pneumonia and tumours among young homosexual men led to the identification of acquired immunodeficiency syndrome (AIDS) and eventually to the discovery of the human immunodeficiency virus (HIV). See also **scan statistic**.

Dispersion: The amount by which a set of observations deviate from their mean. When the values of a set of observations are close to their mean, the dispersion is less than when they are spread out widely from the mean. See also **variance**.

Dispersion parameter: See **generalized linear models**.

Dissimilarity coefficient: A measure of the difference between two observations from (usually) a set of *multivariate data*. For two observations with identical variable values, the dissimilarity is usually defined as zero. See also **metric inequality**.

Dissimilarity matrix: A *square matrix* in which the elements on the main diagonal are zero, and the off-diagonal elements are *dissimilarity coefficients* of each pair of individuals in a set of observations. The elements in such a matrix are usually denoted by δ_{ij}.

Distance measure: See **metric inequality**.

Distributed database: A *database* that consists of a number of component parts which are situated at geographically separate locations.

Distribution-free methods: Statistical techniques of *estimation* and *inference* that are based on a function of the sample observations, the *probability distribution* of which does not depend on a complete specification of the probability distribution of the population from which the sample was drawn. Consequently, the techniques are valid under relatively general assumptions about the underlying population. Often such methods involve only the ranks of the observations rather than the observations themselves. Examples are *Wilcoxon's signed rank test* and *Friedman's two-way analysis of variance*. In many cases these tests are only marginally less powerful than their analogues which assume a particular population distribution (usually a *normal distribution*), even when that assumption is true. Also commonly known as *non-parametric methods*, although the terms are not completely synonymous.

Distribution function: See **probability distribution**.

Divisive methods: *Cluster analysis* procedures that begin with all individuals in a single cluster, which is then successively divided by maximizing some particular measure of the separation of the two resulting clusters. Rarely used in practice. See also **agglomerative hierarchical clustering methods** and **K-means cluster analysis**.

Dixon test: A test for *outliers*. When the sample size (n) is less than or equal to seven, the *test statistic* is

$$r = \frac{y_{(1)} - y_{(2)}}{y_{(1)} - y_{(n)}}$$

where $y_{(1)}$ is the suspected outlier and is the smallest observation in the sample, $y_{(2)}$ is the next smallest and $y_{(n)}$ the largest observation. For $n > 7$, $y_{(3)}$ is used instead of $y_{(2)}$ and $y_{(n-1)}$ instead of $y_{(n)}$. Critical values are available in some statistical tables.

DMF index: A measure, often used in dentistry, that is calculated by adding the number of permanent teeth that are decayed (D), the number that are missing (M), and the number that have been filled (F).

Dorfman scheme: An approach to investigations designed to identify a particular medical condition in a large population, usually by means of a blood test, that may result in a considerable saving in the number of tests carried out. Instead of testing each person separately, blood samples from, say, k people are pooled and analysed together. If the test is negative, this one test clears k people. If the test is positive then each of the k individual blood samples must be tested separately, and in all $k + 1$ tests are required for these k people. If the probability of a positive test (p) is small, the scheme is likely to result in far fewer tests being necessary. For example, if $p = 0.01$, it can be shown that the value of k that minimizes the expected number of tests per person is 11, and that the expected number of tests is 0.2, resulting in 80% saving in the number of tests compared with testing each individual separately.

Dose-ranging trial: A *clinical trial*, usually undertaken at a late stage in the development of a drug, to obtain information about the approprate magnitude of initial and subsequent doses. Most common is the *parallel-dose design*, in which one group of subjects is given a placebo, and other groups different doses of the active treatment.

Dose–response curve: A plot of the values of a response variable against corresponding values of dose of drug received, or level of exposure endured, etc.

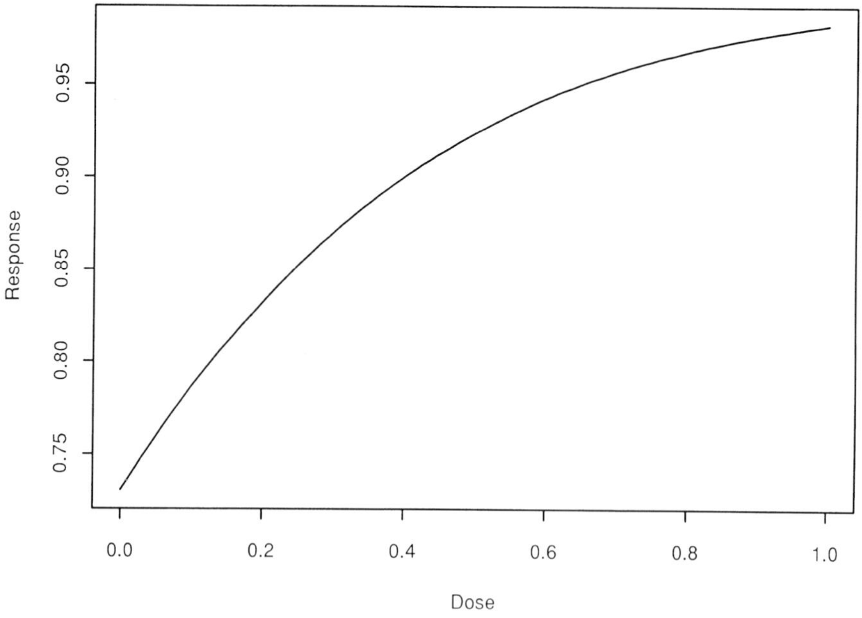

Fig 26 A hypothetical dose–response curve.

Dot plot: A more effective display than a number of other methods, for example, *pie charts* and *bar charts*, for displaying quantitative data which are labelled.

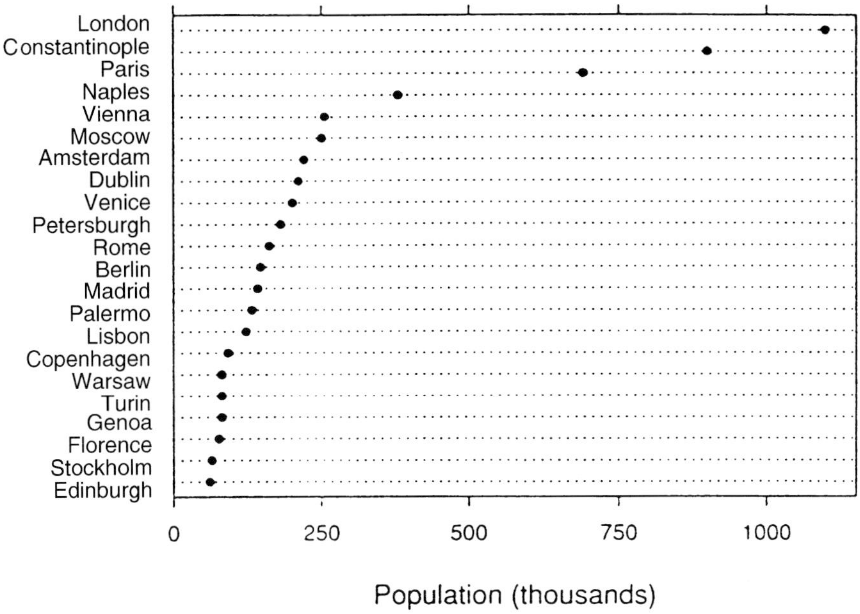

Fig 27 A dot plot giving population size of various cities.

Double-blind: See **blinding**.

Double-centered matrices: Matrices of numerical elements from which both row and column means have been subtracted.

Double-masked: Synonym for **double-blind**.

Double reciprocal plot: A procedure for estimating the parameters in the *Michaelis–Menten* equation, by transforming it to a **Lineweaver–Burk equation**.

Double sampling: A procedure in which, initially, a sample of subjects is selected for obtaining auxiliary information only, and then a second sample is selected in which the variable of interest is observed in addition to the auxiliary information. The second sample is often selected as a subsample of the first. The purpose of this type of sampling is to obtain better estimators by using the relationship between the auxiliary variables and the variable of interest.

Doubling time: A term used, in describing epidemics, for the time taken for the number of infectives to double.

Doubly censored data: Data involving *survival times* in which the time of the originating event and the failure event may both be *censored observations*.

Such data can arise when the originating event is not directly observable, but is detected via periodic *screening studies*.

Doubly multivariate data: A term used for the data collected in those *longitudinal studies* in which more than a single response variable is recorded for each subject on each occasion.

Doubly ordered contingency tables: *Contingency tables* in which both the row and column categories follow a natural order. An example is drug toxicity ranging from mild to severe, against drug dose grouped into a number of classes.

Draughtsman's plot: An arrangement of the pairwise *scatter diagrams* of the variables in a set of *multivariate data* in the form of a square grid. Such an arrangement may be extremely useful in the initial examination of the data. (See Fig. 28 opposite.)

Drift: A term used for the progressive change in assay results throughout an assay run.

Drift parameter: See **Brownian motion**.

Dropout: A patient who withdraws from a study for whatever reason, which may or may not be known. The fate of patients who drop out of an investigation must be determined whenever possible. See also **attrition** and **missing values**.

Dummy variables: The variables resulting from recoding *categorical variables* with more than two categories into a series of *binary variables*. Marital status, for example, if originally labelled 1 for married, 2 for single and 3 for divorced, widowed or separated, could be redefined in terms of two variables as follows

Variable 1: 1 if single, 0 otherwise;
Variable 2: 1 if divorced, widowed or separated, 0 otherwise;

For a married person both new variables would be zero. In general a categorical variable with k categories would be recoded in terms of $k-1$ dummy variables. Such recoding is used before *polychotomous variables* are used as explanatory variables in a *regression analysis*, to avoid the unreasonable assumption that the original numerical codes for the categories, i.e., the values $1, 2, \cdots, k$, correspond to an *interval scale*.

Duncan's multiple range test: A modified form of the *Newman–Keuls multiple comparison test*.

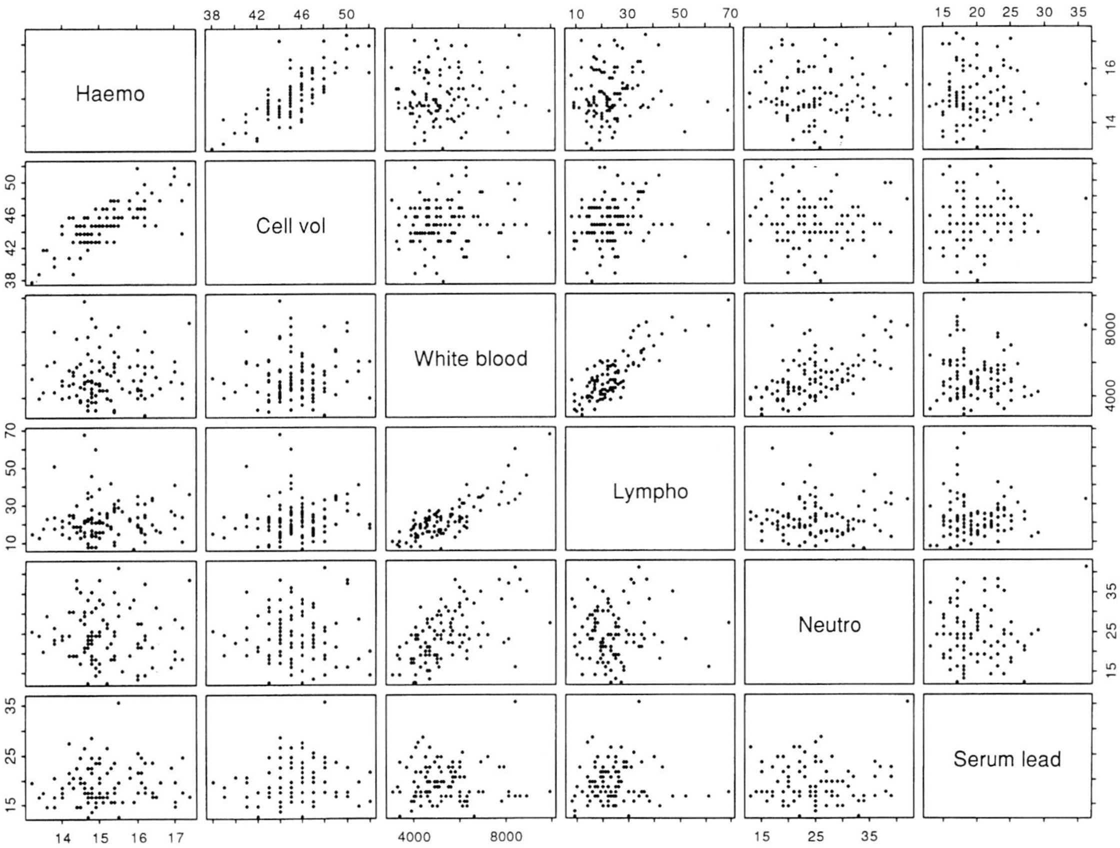

Fig 28 Draughtsman's plot of haemotology variables.

Dunnett's test: A *multiple comparison test* intended for comparing each of a number of treatments with a single control.

Dunn's test: A *multiple comparison test* based on the *Bonferroni test.*

Duplicate data entry: Entering data on to a *database* more than once and comparing results in an effort to record observations as accurately as possible. See also **data editing**.

Duration time: The time that elapses before an epidemic ceases.

Durbin–Watson test: A test that the residuals from a *linear regression* or *multiple regression* are independent. The *test statistic* is

$$D = \frac{\sum_{i=2}^{n}(r_i - r_{i-1})^2}{\sum_{i=1}^{n} r_i^2}$$

where $r_i = y_i - \hat{y}_i$, and y_i and $\hat{y}_i$ are, respectively, the observed and predicted values of the response variable for individual i. D becomes smaller as the *serial correlations* increase. *Critical values* are available in many standard statistical tables.

Dynamic population: A population that gains and loses members.

E

E: Abbreviation for **expected value**.

Ecological statistics: Procedures for studying the dynamics of natural communities and their relation to environmental variables.

EDA: Abbreviation for **exploratory data analysis**.

ED50: Abbreviation for **median effective dose**.

Effect: Generally used for the change in a response variable produced by a change in one or more explanatory variables.

Effective sample size: The sample size after dropouts, deaths and other specified exclusions from the original sample.

Efficacy: The effect of treatment relative to a control, in the ideal situation where all persons fully comply with the treatment regimen to which they were assigned by *random allocation*.

Efficiency: A term applied in the context of comparing different methods of estimating the same parameter; the estimate with lowest variance being regarded as the most efficient. Also used when comparing competing experimental designs, with one design being more efficient than another if it can achieve the same precision with fewer resources.

EGRET: Acronym for the Epidemiological, Graphics, Estimation and Testing program developed for the analysis of data from studies in *epidemiology*. Can be used for *logistic regression*, and models may include *random effects* to allow *overdispersion* to be modelled. The *beta-binomial distribution* can also be fitted.

Ehrenberg's equation: An equation linking the height and weight of children between the ages of 5 and 13, and given by

$$\log \bar{w} = 0.8\bar{h} + 0.4$$

where $\bar{w}$ is the mean weight in kilograms and $\bar{h}$ the mean height in metres. The relationship has been found to hold in England, Canada and France.

Eigenvalues: The roots, $\lambda_1, \lambda_2, \cdots, \lambda_q$, of the qth order polynomial defined by

$$|\mathbf{A} - \lambda\mathbf{I}|$$

where $\mathbf{A}$ is a $q \times q$ *square matrix* and $\mathbf{I}$ is the *identity matrix* of order q. Associated with each root is a non-zero vector, $\mathbf{z}_i$, satisfying

$$\mathbf{A}\mathbf{z}_i = \lambda_i \mathbf{z}_i$$

and $\mathbf{z}_i$ is known as an *eigenvector* of $\mathbf{A}$. Both eigenvalues and eigenvectors appear frequently in accounts of techniques for the analysis of *multivariate data*, such as *principal components analysis* and *factor analysis.* In such methods, eigenvalues usually give the variance of a *linear function* of the variables, and the elements of the eigenvector define a linear function of the variables with a particular property.

Eigenvector: See **eigenvalue**.

Electronic mail (email): The use of computer systems to transfer messages between users; it is usual for messages to be held in a central store for retrieval at the user's convenience.

Email: Abbreviation for **electronic mail.**

EM algorithm: An iterative *algorithm* particularly important in *maximum likelihood estimation* applied in the context of incomplete data problems. The algorithm consists of two steps, known as the E, or Expectation step and the M, or Maximization step. In the former, the *expected value* of the *log-likelihood*, conditional on the observed data and the current estimates of the parameters, is found. In the M-step, this function is maximized to give updated parameter estimates that increase the *likelihood.* The two steps are alternated until convergence is achieved. The algorithm may, in some cases, be very slow to converge. See also **finite mixture distribution** and **imputation**.

Empirical: Based on observation or experiment rather than deduction from basic laws or theory.

Empirical Bayes method: A procedure in which the *prior distribution*, needed in the application of *Bayesian inference*, is determined from empirical evidence.

Endogenous variable: A term primarily used in econometrics to describe those variables which are an inherent part of a system. In most respects, such variables are equivalent to the response or dependent variable in other areas. See also **exogeneous variable**.

Endpoint: A clearly defined outcome or event associated with an individual in a medical investigation. A simple example is the death of a patient.

Entropy: A measure of amount of information received or output by some system, usually given in *bits*.

Entropy measure: A measure, H, of the *dispersion* of a categorical *random variable*, Y, that assumes the integral values $j, 1 \leq j \leq s$, with probability p_j, given by

$$H = -\sum_{j=1}^{s} p_j \log p_j$$

See also **concentration measure**.

Environmental statistics: Procedures for determining how quality of life is affected by the environment, in particular by such factors as air and water pollution, solid wastes, hazardous substances, foods and drugs.

Epidemic chain: See **chains of infection**.

Epidemic curve: A plot of the number of cases of a disease against time. A large and sudden rise corresponds to an epidemic.

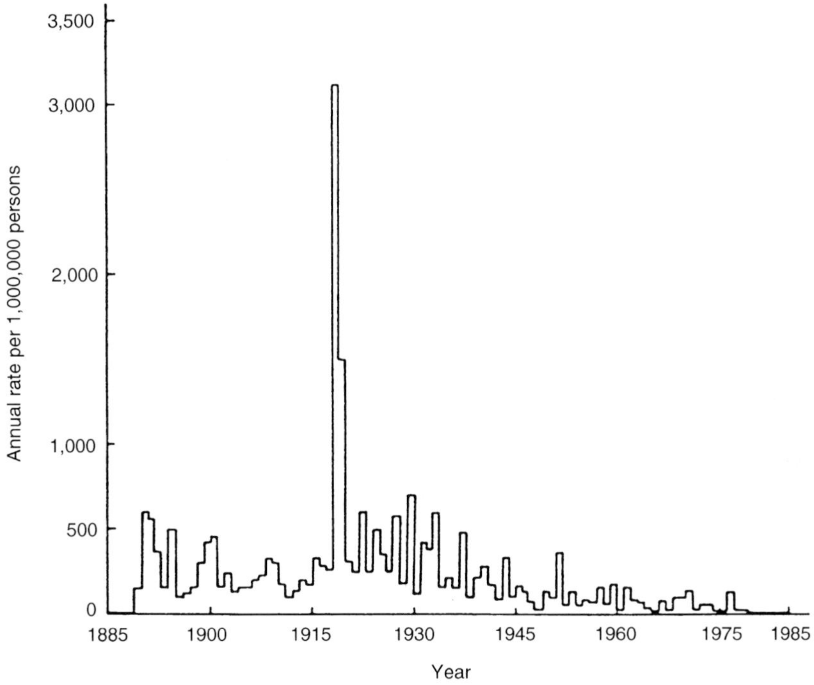

Fig 29 Epidemic curve: influenza mortality in England and Wales 1885–1985.

Epidemic model: A model for the spread of an epidemic in a population.

Epidemiology: The study of the distribution and size of disease problems in human populations, in particular to identify aetiological factors in the pathogenesis of disease, and to provide the data essential for the management, evaluation and planning of services for the prevention, control and treatment of disease. See also **incidence, prevalence, prospective study** and **retrospective study**.

EPILOG PLUS: A command-drive statistical package for epidemiological and *clinical trials* applications. It is structured as a collection of procedures with facilities to carry out many common epidemiological and *survival time* analyses.

Episodic hormone data: Data arising from endocrinology studies involving repeated measurements of blood hormone concentrations over time. Such data usually display a characteristic pattern of episodic pulses, which are produced in response to a burst of neural activity in the hypothalamous. See also **Harris and Stevens forecasting**.

Epistatic genetic variance: The variance of a characteristic that can be explained by the interaction between genes at different loci.

EQS: A software package for fitting *structural equation models*. See also **LISREL**.

Equipotent dose: The dose of a new drug that leads to a response just as effective as the established dose of an old drug.

Equivalent dose: Synonym for **equipotent dose**.

Ergodicity: A property of many time dependent processes, such as certain *Markov chains*, namely, that the eventual distribution of states of the system is independent of the initial state.

Erlangian distribution: A *gamma distribution* with integer parameter values. Arises as the time to the νth event in a *Poisson process*.

Error mean square: See **mean squares**.

Error rate: The proportion of subjects misclassified by a *classification rule* derived from a *discriminant analysis*.

Errors-in-variables problem: See **regression dilution**.

Errors of classification: A term most often used in the context of *retrospective studies*, where it is recognised that a certain proportion of the controls may be at an early stage of disease and should have been diagnosed as cases. Additionally, misdiagnosed cases might be included in the disease group. Both errors lead to underestimates of the *relative risk*.

Errors of the third kind: Giving the right answer to the wrong question!

Estimate: Either a single number (*point estimate*) or a range of numbers (*interval estimate*) which are inferred to be plausible values for some parameter of interest.

Estimation: The process of providing a numerical value for a population parameter on the basis of information collected from a sample. If a single figure is calculated for the unknown parameter, the process is called *point estimation*. If an interval is calculated within which the parameter is likely to fall, then the procedure is called *interval estimation*. See also **least squares estimation, maximum likelihood estimation** and **confidence interval**.

Estimator: A statistic used to provide an estimate for a parameter. The sample mean, for example, is an *unbiased* estimator of the population mean.

Etiological fraction: Synonym for **attributable risk**.

Euclidean distance: For two observations $\mathbf{x}' = [x_1, x_2, \cdots, x_q]$ and $\mathbf{y}' = [y_1, y_2, \cdots, y_q]$ from a set of *multivariate data*, the *distance measure* given by

$$d_{\mathbf{xy}} = \sqrt{\sum_{i=1}^{q} (x_i - y_i)^2}$$

See also **Minkowski distance** and **city-block distance**.

EU model: A model used in investigations of the rate of success of *in vitro* fertilization (IVF), defined in terms of the following two parameters

$$e = \text{Prob(of a viable embryo)}$$
$$u = \text{Prob(of a receptive uterus)}$$

Assuming the two events, viable embryo and receptive uterus, are independent, the probability of observing j implantations out of i transferred embryos is given by

$$P(j|i, u, e) = \binom{i}{j} ue^j (1 - e)^{i-j}, \text{ for } j = 1, 2, 3, \cdots, i.$$

The probability of at least one implantation out of i transferred embryos is given by

$$P(j > 0|i, u, e) = u[1 - (1 - e)^i]$$

and the probability of no implantations by

$$P(j = 0|i, u, e) = 1 - u[1 - (1 - e)^i]$$

The parameters u and e can be estimated by *maximum likelihood estimation* from observations on the number of attempts at IVF with j implantations from i transferred. See also **Barrett and Marshall model for conception**.

Evaluable patients: The patients in a *clinical trial* regarded by the investigator as having satisfied certain conditions and, as a result, retained for the purpose of analysis. Patients not satisfying the required condition are not included in the final analysis.

Event history data: Observations on a collection of individuals, each moving among a small number of states. Of primary interest are the times taken to move between the various states, which are often only incompletely observed because of some form of censoring. The simplest kind of event history data involves *survival times*.

Exogeneous variable: A term primarily used in econometrics to describe those variables that impinge on a system from outside. Essentially equivalent to what are more commonly known as explanatory variables. See also **endogenous variable**.

Expected frequencies: A term usually encountered in the analysis of *contingency tables*. Such frequencies are estimates of the values to be expected under the hypothesis of interest. In a two-dimensional table, for example, the values under independence are calculated from the product of the appropriate row and column totals, divided by the total number of observations.

Expected value (E): The mean of a *random variable*, x, generally denoted as $E(x)$. If the variable is discrete, with *probability distribution* $P(x)$, then $E(x) = \sum_x xP(x)$. If the variable is continuous, the summation is replaced by an integral. The expected value of a function of a random variable, $f(x)$, is defined similarly, i.e.,

$$E(f(x)) = \int_u f(u)g(u)du$$

where $g(x)$ is the probability distribution of x.

Experimental design: The arrangement and procedures used in an *experimental study*. Some general principles of good design are: simplicity, avoidance of *bias*, the use of *random allocation* for forming treatment groups, replication and adequate sample size.

Experimental study: A general term for investigations in which the researcher can deliberately influence events, and investigate the effects of the intervention. *Clinical trials* and many animal studies fall under this heading.

Experimentwise error rate: Synonym for **per-experiment error rate**.

Expert systems: Computer programs designed to mimic the role of an expert human consultant. Such systems are able to cope with the complex problems of medical decision making because of their ability to manipulate symbolic, rather than just numeric, information, and their use of judgemental or heuristic knowledge to construct intelligible solutions to diagnostic problems. Well known examples include the *MYCIN* system, developed at Stanford University, and ABEL, developed at MIT. See also **computer aided diagnosis** and **statistical expert system**.

Explanatory trials: A term sometimes used to describe *clinical trials* that are designed to explain how a treatment works.

Explanatory variables: The variables appearing on the right hand side of the equations defining, for example, *multiple regression* or *logistic regression*, and which seek to predict or 'explain' the response variable. Also commonly known as the *independent variables*, although this is not to be recommended since they are rarely independent of one another.

Exploratory data analysis (EDA): An approach to data analysis that emphasizes the use of informal graphical procedures, not based on prior assumptions about the structure of the data or on formal models for the data. The essence of this approach is that, broadly speaking, data are assumed to possess the following structure

$$\text{Data} = \text{Smooth} + \text{Rough}$$

where the 'Smooth' is the underlying regularity or pattern in the data. The objective of the exploratory approach is to separate the 'Smooth' from the ' Rough' with minimal use of formal mathematics or statistical methods. See also **initial data analysis**.

Exploratory factor analysis: See **factor analyis**.

Exponential distribution: A *probability distribution* of the form

$$f(x) = \lambda e^{-\lambda x}, \qquad x > 0$$

The mean of the distribution is $1/\lambda$ and its variance is $1/\lambda^2$. The exponential is the distribution of intervals between consecutive random events, i.e., those following a *Poisson process*.

Exponential family: A family of *probability distributions* of the form

$$f(x) = \exp\{a(\theta)b(x) + c(\theta) + d(x)\}$$

where θ is a parameter and a, b, c, d are known functions. Includes the *normal distribution, gamma distribution, binomial distribution* and *Poisson distribution* as special cases. The binomial distribution, for example, can be written in the form above as follows:

$$\binom{n}{x} p^x (1-p)^{n-x} = \binom{n}{x} \exp\left\{x \ln \frac{p}{1-p} + n \ln(1-p)\right\}$$

Exponential trend: A *trend*, usually in a *time series*, which is adequately described by an equation of the form $y = ab^x$.

Exposure factor: Synonym for **risk factor**.

Exposure ratio: The ratio of the rates at which persons in the case and control groups of a *retrospective study* are exposed to the *risk factor*.

Extra-binomial variation: A form of **overdispersion**.

Extra period crossover design: The extension of a *crossover design* for a further period not contemplated originally.

Extrapolation: The process of estimating from a data set those values lying beyond the range of the data. In *regression analysis*, for example, a value of the response variable may be estimated from the fitted equation for a new observation having values of the explanatory variables beyond the range of those used in deriving the equation.

Extreme value distribution: The *probability distribution* given by

$$G(x) = 1 - \exp\{-\exp[(x - \alpha)/\beta]\}$$

where α and β are location and scale parameters.

Extreme values: The largest and smallest variate values amongst a sample of observations.

Eyeball test: Informal assessment of data simply by inspection and mental calculation allied with experience of the particular area from which the data arise.

F

Facets: See **generalizability theory**.

Factor: A term used in a variety of ways in statistics, but most commonly to refer to a *categorical variable*, with a small number of levels, under investigation in an experiment as a possible source of variation. Essentially, simply a categorical explanatory variable.

Factor analysis: A procedure that postulates that the correlations or covariances between a set of observed variables, $\mathbf{x}' = [x_1, x_2, \cdots, x_q]$, arise from the relationship of these variables to a small number of underlying, unobservable, *latent variables*, usually known as the *common factors*, $\mathbf{f}' = [f_1, f_2, \cdots, f_k]$, where $k < q$. Explicitly, the model used is

$$\mathbf{x} = \mathbf{\Lambda f} + \mathbf{e}$$

where

$$\mathbf{\Lambda} = \begin{pmatrix} \lambda_{11} & \lambda_{12} & \cdots & \lambda_{1k} \\ \lambda_{21} & \lambda_{22} & \cdots & \lambda_{2k} \\ \vdots & \vdots & \vdots & \vdots \\ \lambda_{q1} & \lambda_{q2} & \cdots & \lambda_{qk} \end{pmatrix}$$

contains the *regression coefficients* (usually known in this context as *factor loadings*) of the observed variables on the common factors. The matrix, $\mathbf{\Lambda}$, is known as the *loading matrix*. The elements of the vector $\mathbf{e}$ are known as *specific variates*. The model implies that the *variance-covariance matrix* of the observed variables, Σ, is of the form

$$\Sigma = \mathbf{\Lambda\Lambda}' + \mathbf{\Psi}$$

where $\mathbf{\Psi}$ is a diagonal matrix containing the variances of the specific variates. A number of approaches are used to estimate the parameters in the model, i.e., the elements of $\mathbf{\Lambda}$ and $\mathbf{\Psi}$, including *maximum likelihood estimation*. After the initial estimation phase, an attempt is generally made to simplify the often difficult task of interpreting the derived factors using a process known as *factor rotation*. In general, the aim is to produce a solution having what is known as *simple structure*, i.e., each common factor affects only a small number of the observed variables. Although based on a well defined model, the method is, in its initial stages at least, essentially exploratory, and such *exploratory factor analysis* needs to be carefully differentiated from *confirmatory factor analysis*, in which a prespecified set of common factors, with some variables constrained to have zero loadings, is tested for consistency with the covariance or correlations of the observed variables. See also **structural equation modelling** and **principal components analysis**.

Factorial designs: Designs which allow two or more questions to be addressed in an investigation. Although used for many years in agriculture and industrial research, such designs have been used only sparingly in medicine. The simplest factorial design is one in which each of two treatments or interventions are either present or absent, so that subjects are divided into four groups; those receiving neither treatment, those having only the first treatment, those having only the second treatment and those receiving both treatments. Such designs enable possible *interactions* between factors to be investigated.

Factor loading: See **factor analysis**.

Factor rotation: The final stage of a *factor analysis*, in which the factors derived initially are transformed to make their interpretation simpler. In general, the aim of the process is to make the common factors more clearly defined, by increasing the size of large factor loadings and decreasing the size of those that are small. *Bipolar factors* are generally split into two separate parts, one corresponding to those variables with positive loadings and the other to those variables with negative loadings. See also **varimax rotation**.

Failure time: Synonym for **survival time**.

False-negative rate: The proportion of cases in which a *diagnostic test* indicates disease absent in patients who have the disease. See also **false-positive rate**.

False-positive rate: The proportion of cases in which a *diagnostic test* indicates disease present in disease-free patients. See also **false-negative rate**.

Familial disease: Disease that exhibits a tendency to familial occurrence due to a variety of possible reasons, for example, genetic, cultural, or common environment.

Familywise error rate: The probability of making any error in a given family of inferences. See also **per-comparison error rate** and **per-experiment error rate**.

Fan-spread model: A term sometimes applied to a model for explaining differences found between naturally occurring groups that are greater than those observed on some earlier occasion; under this model this effect is assumed to arise because individuals who are less unwell, less impaired, etc., and thus score higher initially, may have greater capacity for change or improvement over time.

Fast Fourier transform (FFT): An *algorithm* that finds the *Fourier series* representation of a function accurately and efficiently.

FDA: Abbreviation for **Food and Drug Administration**.

***F*-distribution:** The *probability distribution* of the ratio of two independent *random variables*, each having a *chi-squared distribution*, divided by their respective degrees of freedom. Widely used to assign *P-values* to *mean square ratios* in the *analysis of variance*. The form of the distribution function is that of a *beta distribution* with $\alpha = \nu_1/2$ and $\beta = \nu_2/2$, where ν_1 and ν_2 are the degrees of freedom of the numerator and denominator chi-squared variables, respectively.

Feasibility study: Essentially a synonym for **pilot study**.

Fecundability: The rate at which a sexually active non-contracepting ovulating woman conceives children. In the absence of direct observations on the biological determinants of fecundability, estimators of its distribution are derived from data on waiting times to first conception. See also **EU model**.

Fertility rate: The number of live births in a particular period, expressed as a proportion of potentially fertile women in the population concerned.

FFT: Abbreviation for **fast Fourier transform**.

Fibonacci dose escalation scheme: A scheme designed to estimate the *maximum tolerated dose* during a *Phase I clinical trial*, using as few patients as possible. Using the *National Cancer Institute standards for adverse drug reactions*, the procedure begins patient accrual with three patients at an initial dose level, and continues at each subsequent dose level until at least one toxicity of grade three or above is encountered. Once the latter occurs, three additional patients are entered at that level and six patients are entered into each succeeding level. The search scheme stops when at least two of six patients have toxicities of grade ≥ 3.

Fieller's theorem: A general result that enables *confidence intervals* to be calculated for the ratio of two *random variables* with *normal distributions*.

Finite mixture distribution: A *probability distribution* that results from a *linear function* of a number of component probability distributions. Such distributions are used to model populations thought to contain relatively distinct groups of observations. An early example of the application of such a distribution was that of Pearson in 1894, who applied the following mixture of two *normal distributions* to measurements made on a particular type of crab:

$$f(x) = pN(\mu_1, \sigma_1) + (1 - p)N(\mu_2, \sigma_2)$$

where p is the proportion of the first group in the population, μ_1, σ_1 are, respectively, the mean and standard deviation of the variable in the first group, and μ_2, σ_2 are the corresponding values in the second group. Mixtures of *multivariate normal distributions* are often used as models for *cluster analysis*. See also **NORMIX** and **contaminated normal distribution**.

Finite population: A population of finite size.

Finite population correction: A term sometimes used to describe the extra factor in the variance of the sample mean when n sample values are drawn without replacement from a *finite population* of size N. This variance is given by

$$\text{var}(\bar{x}) = \frac{\sigma^2}{n}\left(1 - \frac{n}{N}\right)$$

the 'correction' term being $(1 - \frac{n}{N})$.

First order autoregressive model: See **autoregressive model**.

First order Markov chain: See **Markov chain**.

First passage time: An important concept in the theory of *stochastic processes*, being the time, T, until the first instant that a system enters a state j, given that it starts in state i.

Fisher's exact test: An alternative procedure to use of the *chi-squared statistic* for assessing the independence of two variables forming a *two-by-two contingency table*, particularly when the *expected frequencies* are small. The method consists of evaluating the sum of the probabilities associated with the observed table and all possible two-by-two tables that have the same row and column totals as the observed data, but exhibit more extreme depature from independence. The probability of each table is calculated from the *hypergeometric distribution*.

Fisher's information matrix: The inverse of the *variance–covariance matrix* of a set of parameters.

Fisher's linear discriminant function: See **discriminant analysis**.

Fisher's z transformation: A transformation of *Pearson's product moment correlation coefficient*, r, given by

$$z = \frac{1}{2}\ln\frac{1+r}{1-r}$$

The statistic z has mean $\frac{1}{2}\ln\frac{1+\rho}{1-\rho}$, where ρ is the population correlation value, and variance $\frac{1}{n-3}$, where n is the sample size. The transformation may be used to test hypotheses and to construct *confidence intervals* for ρ.

Fishing expedition: Synonym for **data dredging**.

Fitted value: Usually used to refer to the value of the response variable as predicted by some estimated model.

Five-number summary: A method of summarizing a set of observations using the minimum value, the lower quartile, the median, upper quartile and maximum value. Forms the basis of the *box-and-whisker plot*.

Five-point assay: A design for a biological assay in which one fifth of the test subjects are allocated to each of two doses of both a standard and a test preparation, the remaining fifth receiving no treatment.

Fixed effects: The effects attributable to a finite set of levels of a factor that are of specific interest. For example, the investigator may wish to compare the effects of three particular drugs on a response variable. *Fixed effects models* are those that contain only factors with this type of effect. See also **random effects**.

Fixed effects model: See **fixed effects**.

Floor effect: See **ceiling effect**.

Flow-chart: A graphical display illustrating the interrelationships between the different components of a system. It acts as a convenient bridge between the conceptualization of a model and the construction of equations.

Folded normal distribution: The *probability distribution* of $z = |x|$, where the *random variable*, x, has a *normal distribution* with zero mean and variance σ^2. Given specifically by

$$f(z) = \frac{1}{\sigma}\sqrt{\frac{2}{\pi}}e^{-z^2/2\sigma^2}$$

Follow-up: The process of locating research subjects or patients to determine whether or not some outcome of interest has occurred.

Food and Drug Administration (FDA): The United States Governmental agency for review and approval of all clinical studies.

Force of mortality: Synonym for **hazard function**.

Forecast: The specific *projection* that an investigator believes is most likely to provide an accurate prediction of a future value of some process.

Forward-looking study: An alternative term for *prospective study*.

Forward selection procedure: See **selection methods in regression**.

Fourfold table: Synonym for **two-by-two contingency table**.

Fourier coefficients: See **Fourier series**.

Fourier series: A series used in the analysis of, generally, a periodic function into its constituent sine waves of different frequencies and amplitudes. The series is

$$\frac{1}{2}a_0 + \sum(a_n \cos nx + b_n \sin nx)$$

where the coefficients are chosen so that the series converges to the function of interest, f; these coefficients (the *Fourier coefficients*) are given by

$$a_n = \frac{1}{\pi}\int_{-\pi}^{\pi} f(x) \cos nx \mathrm{d}x$$
$$b_n = \frac{1}{\pi}\int_{-\pi}^{\pi} f(x) \sin nx \mathrm{d}x$$

for $n = 1, 2, 3, \cdots$. See also **fast Fourier transform.**

Fractal: A term used to describe a geometrical object that continues to exhibit detailed structure over a large range of scales. Snowflakes and coastlines are frequently quoted examples. A medical example is provided by electrocardiograms.

Fractal dimension: A numerical measure of the degree of roughness of a *fractal*. Need not be a whole number, for example, the value for a typical coastline is between 1.15 and 1.25.

Frailty: A term generally used for unobserved individual heterogeneity. Such variation is of major concern in medical statistics, particularly in the analysis of *survival times*, where *hazard functions* can be strongly influenced by selection effects operating in the population. There are a number of possible sources of this heterogeneity, the most obvious of which is that it reflects biological differences, so that, for example, some individuals are born with a weaker heart, or a genetic disposition for cancer. A further possibility is that the heterogeneity arises from the induced weaknesses that result from the stresses of life. Failure to take account of this type of variation may often obscure comparisons between groups, for example, by measures of *relative risk*. A simple model (*frailty model*) which attempts to allow for the variation between individuals is

$$\text{individual hazard function} = Z\lambda(t)$$

where Z is a quantity specific to an individual, considered as a *random variable* over the population of individuals, and $\lambda(t)$ is a basic rate. What is observed, in a population for which such a model holds, is not the individual hazard rate but the net result for a number of individuals with different values of Z.

Frailty model: See **frailty**.

Framingham study: A long-term investigation begun in Framingham, Massachusetts, in 1948, both to identify the relation of possible *risk factors* to the occurrence of chronic circulatory disease and to characterize the natural history of the disease.

Frank's family of bivariate distributions: A class of *bivariate probability distributions* of the form

$$P(X \leq x, Y \leq y) = h_\alpha(x, y) = \log_\alpha\left\{1 + \frac{(\alpha^x - 1)(\alpha^y - 1)}{\alpha - 1}\right\}, \quad \alpha \neq 1$$

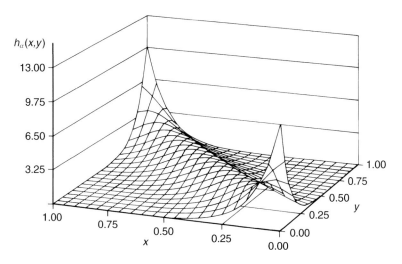

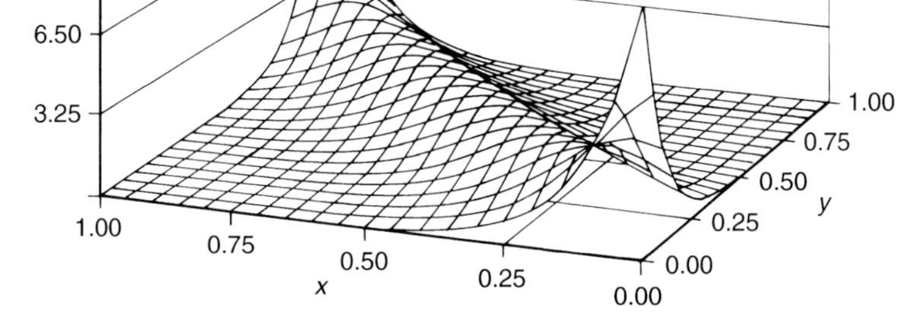

Fig 30 An example of a bivariate distribution from Frank's family.

Freeman–Tukey test: A procedure for assessing the *goodness-of-fit* of some model for a set of data involving counts. The *test statistic* is

$$T = \sum_{i=1}^{k} (\sqrt{O_i} + \sqrt{O_i + 1} - \sqrt{4E_i + 1})^2$$

where k is the number of categories, $O_i, i = 1, 2, \cdots, k$, the observed counts and $E_i, i = 1, 2, \cdots, k$, the *expected frequencies* under the assumed model. The statistic T has asymptotically a *chi-squared distribution* with $k - s - 1$ *degrees of freedom*, where s is the number of parameters in the model. See also **chi-squared statistic** and **likelihood ratio**.

Freeman–Tukey transformation: A transformation of a *random variable*, x, having a *Poisson distribution*, to the form $\sqrt{x} + \sqrt{x+1}$ in order to stabilise its variance.

Frequency distribution: The division of a sample of observations into a number of classes, together with the number of observations in each class. Acts as a useful summary of the main features of the data, such as location, shape and spread. An example of such a table is given below:

Hormone assay values (nmol/L)

Class limits	Observed frequency
75–79	1
80–84	2
85–89	5
90–94	9
95–99	10
100–104	7
105–109	4
110–114	2
$\geq$115	1

See also **histogram**.

Frequency polygon: A diagram used to display graphically the values in a *frequency distribution*. The frequencies are graphed as ordinate against the class mid-points as abscissae. The points are then joined by a series of straight lines. Particularly useful in displaying a number of frequency distributions on the same diagram. (See Fig. 31 opposite.)

Friedman's two-way analysis of variance: A *distribution-free method* that is the analogue of the *analysis of variance* for a design with two factors. Can be applied to data sets that do not meet the assumptions of the parametric approach, namely, normality and homogeneity of variance. Uses only the ranks of the observations.

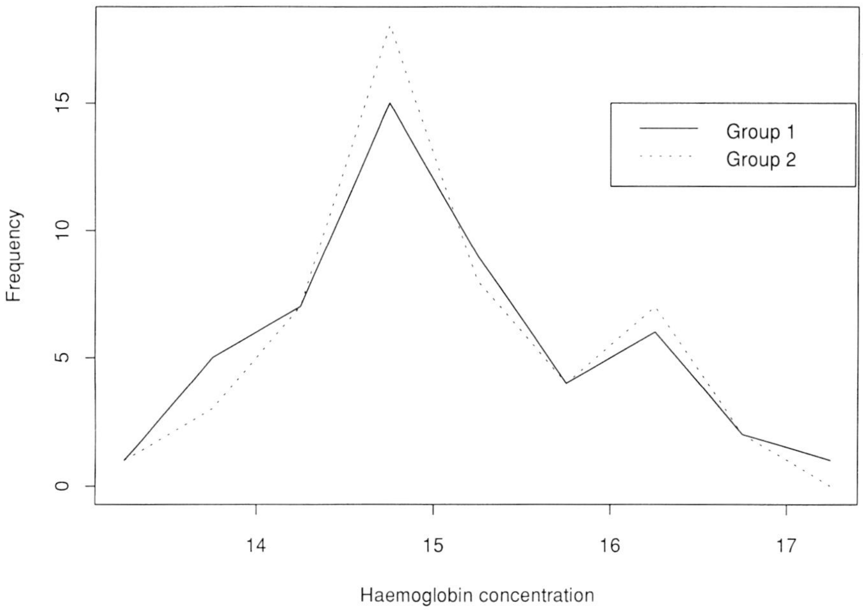

Fig 31 Frequency polygon of haemoglobin concentrations for two groups of men.

Friedman's urn model: An alternative to *random allocation* of patients to treatments in a *clinical trial* with K treatments, that avoids the possible problem of imbalance when the number of available subjects is small. The model considers an urn containing balls of K different colours, and begins with w balls of colour k, $k = 1, \cdots, K$. A draw consists of the following operations:

- select a ball at random from the urn,
- notice its colour k' and return the ball to the urn,
- add to the urn α more balls of colour k' and β more balls of each other colour k, where $k \neq k'$.

Each time a subject is waiting to be assigned to a treatment, a ball is drawn at random from the urn; if its colour is k' then treatment k' is assigned. The values of w, α and β can be any reasonable non-negative numbers. If β is large with respect to α, then the scheme forces the trial to be balanced. The value of w determines the first few stages of the trial. If w is large, more randomness is introduced into the trial; otherwise more balance is enforced.

***F*-test**: A test for the equality of the variances of two populations having *normal distributions*, based on the ratio of the variances of a sample of observations taken from each. Most often encountered in the *analysis of var-*

iance, where testing whether particular variances are the same also tests for the equality of a set of means.

F-to-enter: See **selection methods in regression**.

F-to-remove: See **selection methods in regression**.

Full model: Synonym for **saturated model**.

Functional data analysis: The analysis of data that are functions observed continuously, for example, functions of time.

Functional relationship: The relationship between the 'true' values of variables, i.e., the values assuming that the variables were measured without error. See also **latent variables** and **structural equation modelling**.

Funnel plot: An informal method of assessing the effect of *publication bias*, usually in the context of a *meta-analysis*. The effect measures from each reported study are plotted on the x-axis against, on the y-axis, the corresponding sample sizes. Because of the nature of sampling variability, this plot should, in the absence of publication bias, have the shape of a pyramid with a tapering 'funnel-like' peak. Publication bias will tend to skew the pyramid by selectively excluding studies with small or no significant effects. Such studies predominate when the sample sizes are small, but are increasingly less common as the sample sizes increase. Therefore, their absence removes part of the lower left hand corner of the pyramid. This effect is illustrated in the plots shown opposite.

Future years of life lost: An alternative way of presenting data on mortality in a population, by using the difference between age at death and *life expectancy*.

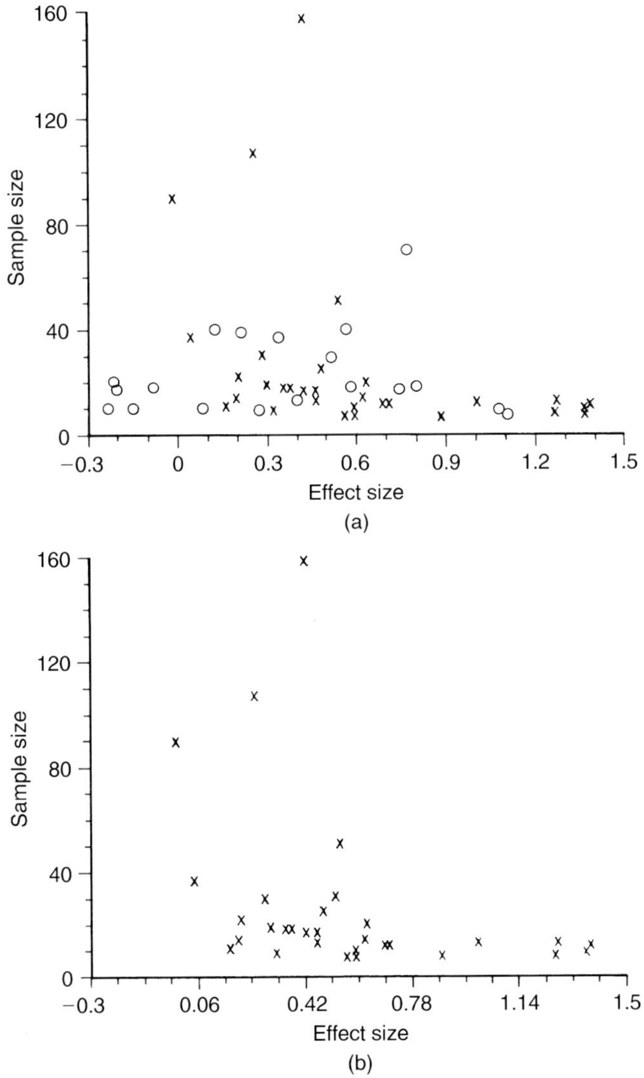

Fig 32 Funnel plot of studies of psychoeducational programs for surgical patients: (a) all studies, (b) published studies only.

G

G²: Symbol for the goodness-of-fit *test statistic* based on the *likelihood ratio*, often used when applying *log-linear models*. Specifically given by

$$G^2 = 2\sum O \ln(O/E)$$

where O and E denote observed and *expected frequencies*. Also used more generally to denote *deviance*.

GAM: Abbreviation for **geographical analysis machine**.

Gambler's fallacy: The belief that if an event has not happened for a long time it is bound to occur soon.

Game theory: The branch of mathematics that deals with the theory of contests between two or more players under specified sets of rules. The subject assumes a statistical aspect when part of the game proceeds under a chance scheme.

Gamma distribution: A *probability distribution* having the form

$$f(x) = \frac{x^{\alpha-1}e^{-x}}{\Gamma(\alpha)}, \qquad x > 0$$

where Γ is the *gamma function*. The mean and variance of the distribution are both equal to the parameter α. (See Fig. 33 opposite.)

Gamma function: The function Γ defined by

$$\Gamma(r) = \int_0^\infty t^{r-1}e^{-t}dt$$

where $r > 0$ (r need not be an integer). The function is *recursive*, satisfying the relationship

$$\Gamma(r+1) = r\Gamma(r)$$

Garbage in garbage out: A term that draws attention to the fact that sensible output only follows from sensible input. Specifically, if the data is originally of dubious quality then so also will be the results.

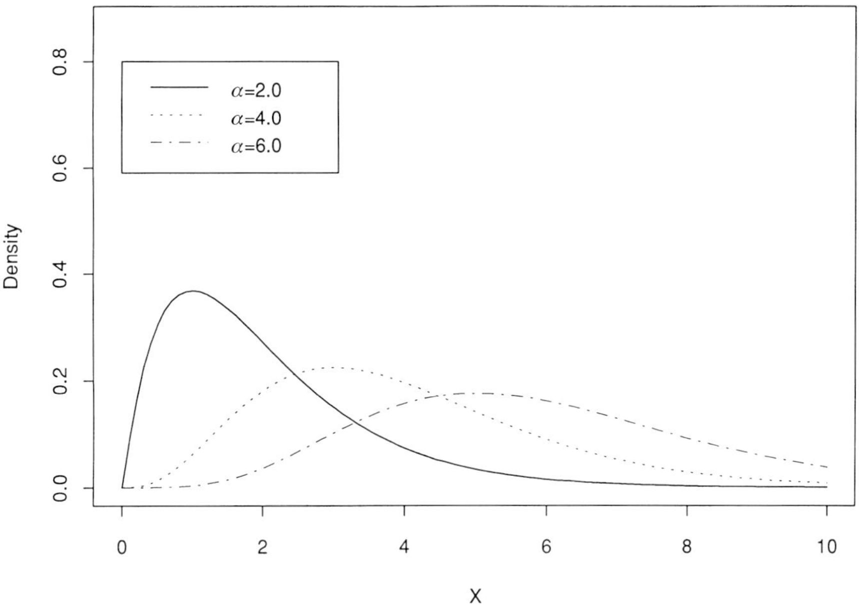

Fig 33 Gamma distributions for a number of parameter values.

GAUSS: A high level programming language with extensive facilities for the manipulation of matrices.

Gaussian distribution: Synonym for **normal distribution**.

Gaussian quadrature: A procedure for performing numerical integration (or quadrature) using a series expansion of the form

$$\int f(x)\phi(x)\mathrm{d}x \approx \sum_{i=1}^{m} w_m f(x_m)$$

where x_m are the Gaussian quadrature points and w_m the associated weights, both of which are available from tables.

Gauss–Markov theorem: A theorem that proves that if the error terms in a *multiple regression* model have the same variance and are uncorrelated, then the estimates of the parameters in the model produced by *least squares estimation* are better (in the sense of having lower dispersion about the mean) than those given by any other *unbiased linear estimator*.

Geary's ratio: A test of normality, in which the *test statistic* is

$$G = \frac{\text{mean deviation}}{\text{standard deviation}}$$

In samples from a *normal distribution*, G tends to $\sqrt{\frac{2}{\pi}}$ as n tends to infinity. Aims to detect depatures from *mesokurtosis* in the parent population.

GEE: Abbreviation for **generalized estimating equations**.

Gehan's generalized Wilcoxon test: A *distribution-free method* for comparing the *survival times* of two groups of individuals. See also **Cox–Mantel test**.

Gene frequency: For a given population, the number of loci at which a given *allele* is found, divided by the total number of loci at which it could occur.

General health questionnaire (GHQ): A self-administered questionnaire used for detecting individuals suffering from non-psychotic psychiatric illness. Consists of thirty questions about current symptoms, abnormal feelings and thoughts, and aspects of observable behaviour. The thirty items are scored as *binary variables* and summed to provide an overall score. The properties of the instrument have been carefully explored and it has been widely used in psychiatric *epidemiology*.

Generalizability theory: A theory of measurement that recognises that in any measurement situation there are multiple (in fact infinite) sources of variation (called *facets* in the theory), and that an important goal of measurement is to attempt to identify and measure *variance components* which are contributing error to an estimate. Strategies can then be implemented to reduce the influence of these sources on the measurement.

Generalized additive models: Models which use *smoothing* techniques, such as *locally weighted regression* and *lowess*, to identify and represent possible non-linear relationships between the explanatory and response variables, as an alternative to considering polynomial terms or searching for the appropriate transformations of both response and explanatory variables. With these models, the *link function* of the *expected value* of the response variable is modelled as the sum of a number of smooth functions of the explanatory variables, rather than in terms of the explanatory variables themselves. See also **generalized linear models**.

Generalized distance: See **Mahalanobis** $\mathbf{D^2}$.

Generalized estimating equations (GEE): An extension of *generalized linear models* that provides a unified and flexible approach to the analysis of data from a *longitudinal study*. Of particular relevance when the repeated measurements are *binary variables* or counts, and a number of possibly *time dependent covariates* are also measured. In such cases the main problem is that of modelling the possible correlations among the repeated observations for a given subject. The *likelihood* is often intractable and involves many *nuisance parameters* in addition to those of main concern. Consequently a *quasi-likelihood* approach is adopted.

Generalized linear models (GLM): A class of models that arise from a natural generalization of ordinary *linear regression*. Here some function (the *link function*) of the *expected value* of the response variable, y, is modelled as a linear combination of the explanatory variables, $x_1, x_2, \cdots, x_q$, i.e.,

$$f(E(y)) = \beta_0 + \beta_1 x_1 + \beta_2 x_2 + \cdots + \beta_q x_q$$

where f is the link function. The other components of such models are a specification of the form of the variance of the response variable and of its *probability distribution*. Particular types of model arise from this general formulation by specifying the appropriate link function, variance and distribution. For example, *multiple regression* corresponds to an identity link function, constant variance and a *normal distribution*. *Logistic regression* arises from a *logit* link function and a *binomial distribution*; here the variance of the response is related to its mean as variance $=$ mean$(1 - \frac{\text{mean}}{n})$, where n is the number of observations. A *dispersion parameter* (often also known as a *scale factor*), can also be introduced to allow for a phenomenon such as *overdispersion*. For example, if the variance is greater that would be expected from a binomial distribution, then it could be specified as $\phi\,\text{mean}(1 - \frac{\text{mean}}{n})$. In most applications of such models the scaling factor, ϕ, will be unity. Estimates of the parameters in such models are generally found by *maximum likelihood estimation*. See also **GLIM**, **generalized additive models** and **generalized estimating equations**.

Generalized P values: A procedure introduced to deal with those situations where it is difficult or impossible to derive a significance test because of the presence of *nuisance parameters*.

Generalized variance: An analogue of the variance for use with *multivariate data*. Given by the *determinant* of the *variance–covariance matrix* of the observations.

Genetic distance: A *distance measure* used by geneticists when describing groups or populations in terms of *gene frequencies*. Specifically defined as

$$d_{AB} = (1 - \cos\theta)^{\frac{1}{2}}$$

where

$$\cos\theta = \sum_i (p_{iA} p_{iB})^{\frac{1}{2}}$$

The terms p_{iA} and p_{iB} are the gene frequencies for the *i*th *allele* at a given locus in the two populations.

Genetic epidemiology: The analysis of the familial distributions of traits, with a view to understanding any possible genetic basis, by disentangling, as far as possible, environmental and genetic causes.

Genotype: The genetic constitution of an organism, i.e., what *alleles* it has, as distinguished from its physical appearance (its *phenotype*).

GENSTAT: A general purpose piece of statistical software for the management and analysis of data. The package incorporates a wide variety of data handling procedures and a wide range of statistical techniques, including *regression analysis, cluster analysis*, and *principal components analysis.* Its use as a sophisticated statistical programming language enables non-standard methods of analysis to be implemented relatively easily.

Geographical analysis machine (GAM): A procedure designed to detect clusters of rare diseases in a particular region. Circles of fixed radii are created at each point of a square grid covering the study region. Neighbouring circles are allowed to overlap to some fixed extent and the number of cases of the disease within each circle counted. Significance tests are then performed, based on the total number of cases and on the number of individuals at risk, both in total and in the circle in question, during a particular census year. See also **scan statistic**.

Geographical correlations: The correlations between variables measured as averages over geographical units.

Geometric distribution: The *probability distribution* of the number of trials until the first 'success' in a series of *random variables* from a *Bernoulli distribution.* Specifically, the distribution is given by

$$f(x) = p(1-p)^{x-1}, \qquad x = 1, 2, \cdots$$

where p is the probability of a success. The mean of the distribution is $1/p$ and the variance is $(1-p)/p^2$.

Geometric mean: A measure of location, g, calculated from a set of observations, $x_1, x_2, \cdots, x_n$, as

$$g = \left(\prod_{j=1}^{n} x_j\right)^{\frac{1}{n}}$$

GHQ: Abbreviation for **general health questionnaire**.

Gibbs sampling: A technique widely used in image processing for the restoration of blurred or distorted pictures. In statistics, the procedure is used for calculating numerical estimates of *marginal probability distributions*, primarily in the context of making *Bayesian inferences* in a wide class of *generalized linear models* and *Cox's proportional hazards models*. Using the method in this way avoids the computational problems of the direct numerical integration of the *posterior distribution* to obtain the required marginal distributions of parameters of interest. Essentially, the procedure provides samples from a *joint distribution* via iterated sampling from a series of *conditional distributions* that are often of familiar form, such as *normal distributions* or *gamma distributions*. The procedure succeeds because it reduces the problem of dealing simultaneously with a large number of intricately related unknown parameters and missing data into a much simpler problem of dealing with one unknown quantity at a time, sampling each from its conditional distribution. See also **data augmentation**.

GLIM: A software package particularly suited for fitting *generalized linear models* (the acronym stands for Generalized Linear Interactive Modelling), including *log-linear models*, *logistic models*, and models based on the *complementary log-log transformation*. A large number of GLIM macros are now available that can be used for a variety of non-standard statistical analyses.

GLM: Abbrevation for **generalized linear model**.

Glyphs: A graphical representation of *multivariate data*, in which each observation is represented by a circle, with rays of different lengths indicating the

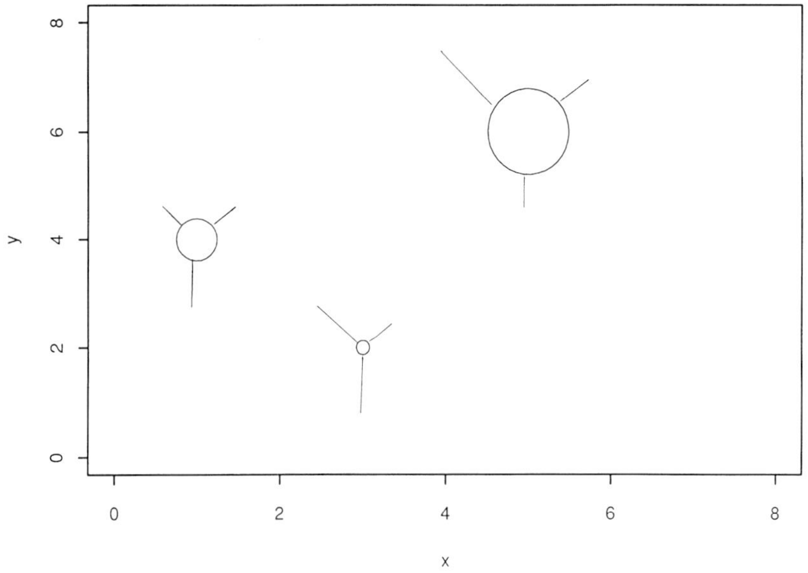

Fig 34 An example of glyphs.

values of the observed variables. See also **Andrews' plots** and **Chernoff's faces.**

Gold standard trials: Usually used for *clinical trials* which involve a new therapy, a standard therapy and a placebo.

Gompertz curve: A curve used to describe the size of a population (y) as a function of time (t), where relative growth rate declines at a constant rate. Explicitly given by

$$y = ae^{-b^t}$$

Goodman–Kruskal measures of association: A series of indices for measuring the strength of the association between the two variables forming a *contingency table*. Each measure is designed for a specific class of problem. In particular, different indices are used for unordered and ordered variables, and for situations in which one variable may be considered explanatory and the other the response.

Goodness-of-fit statistics: Measures of the agreement between a set of sample observations and the corresponding values predicted from some model of interest. Many such measures have been suggested; see *chi-squared statistic, deviance, likelihood ratio,* G^2 and X^2.

Gower's similarity coefficient: A *similarity coefficient* particularly suitable when the measurements contain both *continuous variables* and *categorical variables*.

Grade of membership model: A general *distribution-free method* for the clustering of *multivariate data* in which only *categorical variables* are involved. The model assumes that individuals can exhibit characteristics of more than one cluster, and that the state of an individual can be represented by a set of numerical quantities, each one corresponding to one of the clusters, that measure the 'strength' or grade of membership of the individual for the cluster. Estimation of these quantities and the other parameters in the model is undertaken by *maximum likelihood estimation.* See also **latent class analysis.**

Graeco–Latin square: An extension of a *Latin square* that allows for three extraneous sources of variation in an experiment. A three-by-three example of such a square is

Aα	Bβ	Cγ
Bγ	Cα	Aβ
Cβ	Aγ	Bα

Grand mean: Mean of all the values in a grouped data set irrespective of groups.

Graphical methods: A generic term for those techniques in which the results are given in the form of a graph, diagram or some other form of visual display. Examples are *Andrew's plots*, *Chernoff's faces* and *coplots*.

Graph theory: A branch of mathematics concerned with the properties of sets of points (vertices or nodes) some of which are connected by lines known as edges. A *directed graph* is one in which direction is associated with the edges and an *undirected graph* is one in which no direction is involved in the connections between points. See also **conditional independence graph**.

Greatest characteristic root test: Synonym for **Roy's largest root criterion**.

Greenhouse–Geisser correction: A method of adjusting the degrees of freedom of the within subject *F-tests* in the *analysis of variance* of *longitudinal data*, so as to allow for possible departures of the *variance–covariance matrix* of the measurements from the assumption of *sphericity*. If this condition holds for the data, then the correction factor is unity and the simple F-tests are valid. Departures from sphericity result in an estimated correction factor less than unity, thus reducing the degrees of freedom of the relevant F-tests. See also **Huynh–Feldt correction**.

Greenwood's formula: A formula giving the variance of the *product limit estimator* of a *survival function*, namely

$$\text{var}(\hat{S}(t)) = [\hat{S}(t)]^2 \sum_{t_{(r)} \leq t} \frac{d_j}{r_j(r_j - d_j)}$$

where $\hat{S}(t)$ is the estimated survival function at time t, $t_{(1)} < t_{(2)} < \cdots < t_{(n)}$ are the ordered, observed *survival times*, r_j is the number of individuals at risk at time t_j, and d_j is the number who experience the event of interest at time t_j. (Individuals censored at t_j are included in r_j.)

Grouped binary data: Observations on a *binary variable* tabulated in terms of the proportion of one of the two possible outcomes amongst patients or subjects who have, for example, the same diagnosis or same sex.

Grouped data: Data recorded as frequencies of observations in particular intervals.

Group sequential design: See **sequential analysis**.

Growth charts: Synonym for **centile reference charts**.

Growth curve: An expression giving either the size of a population or the size of an individual as a function of time. See also **Gompertz curve**.

Growth rate: A measure of population growth, calculated as

$$\frac{\text{live births during the year} - \text{deaths during the year}}{\text{midyear population}} \times 100$$

Grubb's estimators: Estimators of the measuring precisions when two instruments or techniques are used to measure the same quantity. For example, if the two measurements are denoted by x_i and y_i for $i = 1, \cdots n$, and we assume that

$$x_i = \tau_i + \epsilon_i$$
$$y_i = \tau_i + \delta_i$$

where τ_i is the correct unknown value of the ith quantity and ϵ_i and δ_i are measurement errors assumed to be independent, then Grubb's estimators are

$$\hat{V}(\tau_i) = \text{covariance}(x, y)$$
$$\hat{V}(\epsilon_i) = \text{variance}(x) - \text{covariance}(x, y)$$
$$\hat{V}(\delta_i) = \text{variance}(y) - \text{covariance}(x, y)$$

Guarantee time: See **two-parameter exponential distribution**.

Gumbel distribution: An asymmetric *probability distribution* encountered in some versions of *Cox's proportional hazards model*, and given by

$$f(x) = \frac{1}{\kappa} e^{(x-\alpha)/\kappa} \exp(-e^{(x-\alpha)/\kappa})$$

where α and κ are unknown parameters. See also **extreme value distribution** and **complementary log-log transformation**.

H

H_0: Symbol for **null hypothesis**.

H_1: Symbol for **alternative hypothesis**.

Haldane's estimator: An estimator of the *odds ratio*, given by

$$\hat{\psi} = \frac{(a+\frac{1}{2})(d+\frac{1}{2})}{(b+\frac{1}{2})(c+\frac{1}{2})}$$

where a, b, c and d are the cell frequencies in the *two-by-two contingency table* of interest. See also **Jewell's estimator**.

Half-normal plot: A plot for diagnosing model inadequacy or revealing the presence of *outliers*, in which the absolute values of, for example, the *residuals* from a *multiple regression* are plotted against the quantiles of the *standard normal distribution*. Outliers will appear at the top right of the plot as points that are separated from the others, while systematic departures from a straight line could indicate that the model is unsatisfactory.

Halo effect: The tendency of a subject's performance on some task to be overrated because of the observer's perception of the subject 'doing well' gained in an earlier exercise or when assessed in a different area.

Hanging rootogram: A diagram comparing an observed *rootogram* with a fitted curve, in which differences between the two are displayed in relation to the horizontal axis, rather than to the curve itself. This makes it easier to spot large differences and to look for patterns. (See Fig. 35 overleaf.)

HAQ: Abbreviation for **health assessment questionnaire**.

Hardy–Weinberg law: The law stating that both *gene frequencies* and *genotype* frequencies will remain constant from generation to generation in an infinitely large interbreeding population in which mating is at random and there is no selection, migration or mutation. In a situation where a single pair of *alleles* (A and a) is considered, the frequencies of germ cells carrying A and a are defined as p and q respectively. At equilibrium the frequencies of the genotype classes are $p^2(AA)$, $2pq(Aa)$ and $q^2(aa)$.

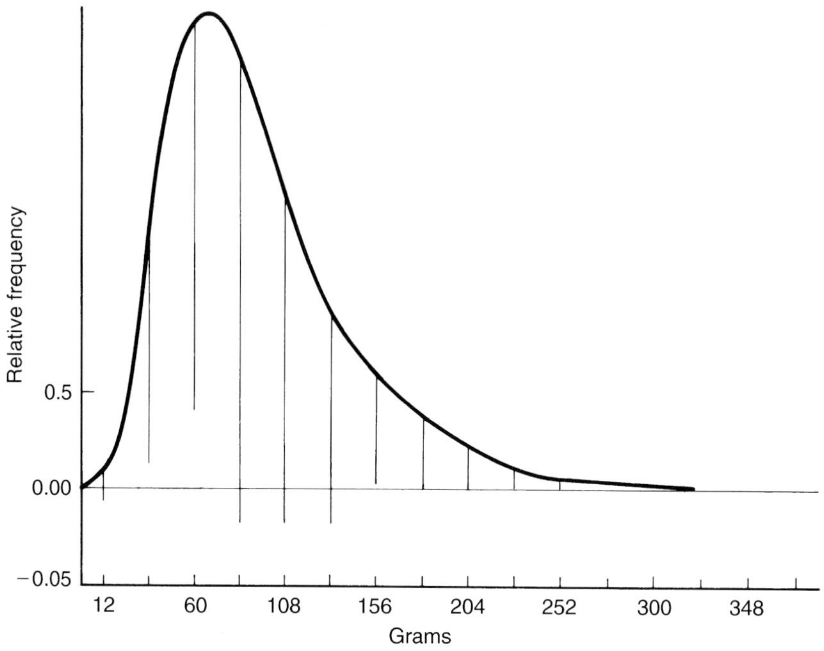

Fig 35 An example of a hanging rootogram.

Harmonic analysis: The representation of a *time series* by a sum of trigonometric terms of varying period and amplitude, for example, a *Fourier series*. Generally used both to smooth the series and to help in the identification of important periodic components. See also **periodogram** and **spectral analysis**.

Harmonic mean: The reciprocal of the arithmetic mean of the reciprocals of a set of observations $x_1, x_2, \cdots, x_n$. Specifically obtained from the equation

$$\frac{1}{H} = \frac{1}{n}\sum_{i=1}^{n}\frac{1}{x_i}$$

Used in some methods of analysing *non-orthogonal designs*. The harmonic mean is either smaller than or equal to the arithmetic mean.

Harris and Stevens forecasting: A method of making short term forecasts in a *time series* that is subject to abrupt changes in pattern and transient effects. Examples of such series are those arising from measuring the concentration of certain biochemicals in biological organisms, or the concentration of plasma growth hormone. The changes are modelled by adding a random perturbation vector having zero mean to a linearly updated parameter vector. See also **episodic hormone data**.

Hartley's test: A simple test of the equality of variances of the populations corresponding to the groups in a *one way design*. The *test statistic* (if each group has the same number of observations) is the ratio of the largest (s^2 largest) to the smallest (s^2 smallest) within group variance, i.e.,

$$F = \frac{s^2 \text{ largest}}{s^2 \text{ smallest}}$$

Critical values are available in many statistical tables. The test is sensitive to departures from normality. See also **Bartlett's test** and **Box's test**.

Hat matrix: A matrix, **H**, arising in *multiple regression*, which gives the predicted value of the response variable corresponding to each observed value via the equation

$$\hat{\mathbf{y}} = \mathbf{H}\mathbf{y}$$

H is a *symmetric matrix* and is also *idempotent*. The diagonal elements of **H** are useful diagnostically in assessing the results from the analysis.

Hausdorf dimension: Synonym for **fractal dimension**.

Hawthorne effect: A term used for the effect that might be produced in an experiment simply from the awareness by the subjects that they are participating in some form of scientific investigation. The name comes from a study of industrial efficiency at the Hawthorne Plant in Chicago in the 1920s.

Hazard function: The probability that an individual experiences an event (death, improvement, etc.) in a small time interval, given that the individual has survived up to the beginning of the interval. It is a measure of how likely an individual is to experience an event, as a function of the age of the individual. The hazard function may remain constant, increase, decrease, or take on some more complex shape. The function can be estimated as the proportion of individuals experiencing an event in an interval per unit time, given that they have survived to the beginning of the interval, that is,

$$\hat{h}(t) = \frac{\text{number of individuals experiencing an event in interval beginning at } t}{(\text{number of individuals surviving at } t)(\text{interval width})}$$

Care is needed in the interpretation of the hazard function, both because of selection effects due to variation between individuals, and variation within each individual over time. For example, individuals with a high risk are more prone to experience an event early, and those remaining at risk will tend to be a selected group with a lower risk. This will result in the hazard rate being 'pulled down' to an increasing extent as time passes. See also **survival function**, **bathtub curve** and **frailty models**.

Hazard regression: A procedure for modelling the *hazard function* that does not depend on the assumptions made in *Cox's proportional hazards model*, namely that the log-hazard function is an additive function of both time and the vector of covariates. In this approach, *spline functions* are used to model the log-hazard function.

Health assessment questionnaire (HAQ): A multidimensional instrument developed by the Stanford Arthritis Centre that measures outcome in terms of mortality, disability, pain, latrogenic events and economic impact. See also **activities of daily living scale**.

Healthy worker effect: The phenomenon whereby employed individuals tend to have lower mortality rates than those unemployed. The effect, which can pose a serious problem in the interpretation of industrial *cohort studies*, has two main components:

- selection at recruitment to exclude the chronically sick, resulting in low *standardized mortality rates* among recent recruits to an industry
- a secondary selection process, by which workers who become unfit during employment tend to leave, again leading to lower standardized mortality ratios amongst long-serving employees.

Hello–goodbye effect: A phenomenon originally described in psychotherapy research, but one which may arise whenever a subject is assessed on two occasions, with some intervention between the visits. Before an intervention a person may present himself/herself in as bad a light as possible, thereby hoping to qualify for treatment, and impressing staff with the seriousness of his/her problems. At the end of the study the person may want to 'please' the staff with his/her improvement, and so may minimize any problems. The result is to make it appear that there has been some improvement when none has occurred, or to magnify the effects that did occur.

Helmert contrast: A *contrast* often used in the *analysis of variance*, in which each level of a factor is tested against the average of the remaining levels. So, for example, if three groups are involved, of which the first is a control, and the other two treatment groups, the first contrast tests the control group against the average of the two treatments and the second tests whether the two treatments differ.

Heritability: A measure of the degree to which a *phenotype* is genetically influenced and can be modified by selection. Specifically given by

$$H = V_a/V_p$$

where V_a = variance due to genes with additive effects, and V_p = the phenotype variance.

Hessian matrix: A $q \times q$ matrix of second partial derivatives of the *log-likelihood* of a model with q parameters.

Heterogeneous: A term used in statistics to indicate the inequality of some quantity of interest (usually a variance) in a number of different groups, populations, etc. See also **homogeneous**.

Heuristic computer program: A computer program which attempts to use the same sort of selectivity in searching for solutions that human beings use.

Heywood cases: Solutions obtained when using *factor analysis* in which one or more of the variances of the *specific variates* become negative.

Hierarchical design: Synonym for **nested design**.

Hierarchical models: A series of models for a set of observations, where each model results from adding or deleting parameters from other models in the series.

Hidden time effects: Effects that arise in data sets that may simply be a result of collecting the observations over a period of time. See also **cusum**.

High breakdown methods: Methods that are designed to be resistant to even multiple severe *outliers*. Such methods are an extreme example of *robust statistics*.

High–medium–low method: A method used in demographic forecasting to quantify uncertainty in projections. High, medium and low sets of assumptions are constructed and projections based on each calculated.

Hinge: A more exotic (but less desirable) term for **quartile**.

HIPE: Abbreviation for **hospital in-patient enquiry**.

Histogram: A graphical representation of a set of observations, in which class frequencies are represented by the areas of rectangles centered on the class interval. If the latter are all equal, the heights of the rectangles are also proportional to the observed frequencies. (See Fig. 36 overleaf.)

Historical controls: A group of patients treated in the past with a standard therapy, used as the control group for evaluating a new treatment on current patients. Although used fairly frequently in medical investigations, the approach is not to be recommended since possible *biases*, due to other factors that may have changed over time, can never be satisfactorily eliminated. See also **literature controls**.

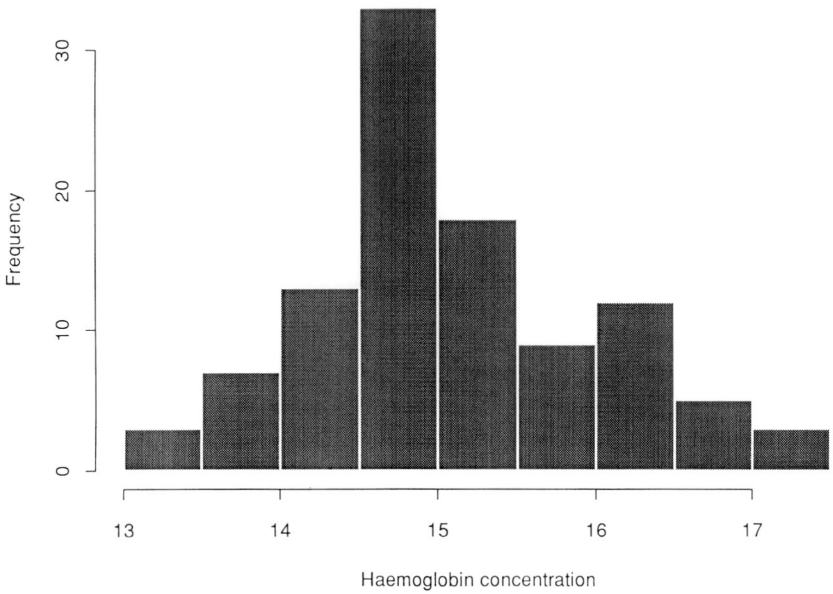

Fig 36 Histogram of haemoglobin concentrations.

Historical prospective studies: A 'prospective study' in which the cohort to be investigated and its subsequent disease history are identified from past records, for example, from information of an individual's work history.

Hit rate: A term occasionally used for the number of correct classifications in a *discriminant analysis*.

Holdover effect: Synonym for **carryover effect**.

Homogeneous: A term that is used in statistics to indicate the equality of some quantity of interest (most often a variance), in a number of different groups, populations, etc. See also **heterogeneous**.

Hospital controls: See **control group**.

Hospital discharge rate: The number of discharges from hospital during a time period, divided by the estimated midyear population for the hospital's catchment area. It is usually expressed per 1000 persons per year.

Hospital in-patient enquiry (HIPE): In England and Wales, the collection of data for every tenth patient discharged from a general hospital. In addition to the age, sex and marital status of the patient, information about date of admission, discharge, time on waiting list, diagnosis and operations undergone, is recorded.

Hot deck: A method of *imputation* in which *missing values* are replaced by values selected from amongst existing cases.

Hotelling–Lawley trace: See **multivariate analysis of variance**.

Hotelling's T^2 test: A generalization of *Student's t-test* for *multivariate data*. Can be used to test either whether the population *mean vector* of a set of q variables is the null vector, or whether the mean vectors of two populations are equal. In the latter case the relevant *test statistic* is calculated as

$$T^2 = \frac{n_1 n_2 (\bar{\mathbf{x}}_1 - \bar{\mathbf{x}}_2)' \mathbf{S}^{-1} (\bar{\mathbf{x}}_1 - \bar{\mathbf{x}}_2)}{n_1 + n_2}$$

where $n_1$and n_2 are sample sizes, $\bar{\mathbf{x}}_1$ and $\bar{\mathbf{x}}_2$ are sample mean vectors, and $\mathbf{S}$ is a weighted average of the separate sample *variance–covariance matrices*. Under the hypothesis that the population mean vectors are the same, $\frac{n_1+n_2-q-1}{(n_1+n_2-2)q} T^2$ has an *F-distribution* with q and $(n_1 + n_2 - q - 1)$ degrees of freedom. See also **Mahalanobis D^2**.

Household survey: A descriptive survey of illness and disability, performed by interviewing persons in their own homes, often by questioning a single informant about other members of the household.

Human capital model: A model for evaluating the economic implication of disease in terms of the economic loss of a person succumbing to morbidity or mortality at some specified age. Often such a model has two components, the direct cost of disease, for example, medical management and treatment, and the indirect cost of disease, namely, the loss of economic productivity due to a person being removed from the labour force.

Human height growth curves: The growth of human height is, in general, remarkably regular, apart from the pubertal growth spurt. A satisfactory longitudinal *growth curve* is extremely useful as it enables long series of measurements to be replaced by a few parameters, and might permit early detection and treatment of growth abnormalities. Several such curves have been proposed, of which perhaps the most successful is the following five parameter curve:

$$X = A - \frac{2(A - B)}{\exp[C(t - E)] + \exp[D(t - E)]}$$

where t = time (age measured from the day of birth), X = height reached at age t, A = adult height, B = height reached by child at age E, C = a first time-scale factor in units of inverse time, D=a second time-scale factor in units of inverse time, E=approximate time at which the pubertal growth spurt occurs.

Huynh–Feldt correction: A correction term applied in the analysis of data from *longitudinal studies* by simple *analysis of variance* procedures, to ensure that the within subject *F-tests* are approximately valid even if the assumption of *sphericity* is invalid. See also **Greenhouse–Geisser correction** and **Mauchly test**.

Hypergeometric distribution: A *probability distribution* associated with *sampling without replacement* from a population of finite size. If the population consists of r elements of one kind and $N - r$ of another, then the probability of finding x elements of the first kind when a *random sample* of size n is drawn is given by

$$P(x) = \frac{\binom{r}{x}\binom{N-r}{n-x}}{\binom{N}{n}}$$

The mean of x is nr/N and its variance is $(\frac{nr}{N})(1 - \frac{r}{n})(\frac{N-n}{N-1})$. When N is large and n is small compared with N, the hypergeometric distribution can be approximated by the *binomial distribution*.

Hypothesis testing: A general term for the procedure of assessing whether sample data is consistent or otherwise with statements made about the population. See also **null hypothesis, alternative hypothesis, composite hypothesis, significance test, significance level, type I** and **type II error**.

I

IBD: Abbreviation for **identical-by-descent**.

IDA: Abbreviation for **initial data analysis**.

Idempotent matrix: A *symmetric matrix*, **A**, with the property that $\mathbf{A} = \mathbf{A}^2$. An example is:

$$\mathbf{A} = \begin{pmatrix} 1 & 0 & 0 \\ 0 & 1 & 0 \\ 0 & 0 & 1 \end{pmatrix}$$

Identical-by-descent (IBD): A term used when two genes at a given locus have both been inherited from a common ancestor. For example, in a family without inbreeding, two siblings who have inherited the same gene from their father but two different genes from their mother have one gene (the paternal one) to which the term applies.

Identification: The degree to which there is sufficient information in the sample observations to estimate the parameters in a proposed model. An *unidentified model* is one in which there are too many parameters in relation to the number of observations to make estimation possible. A *just identified model* corresponds to a *saturated model*. Finally an *overidentified model* is one in which parameters can be estimated, and there remain some degrees of freedom to allow the fit of the model to be assessed.

Identity matrix: A diagonal matrix in which all the elements on the leading diagonal are unity and all other elements are zero.

Ill conditioned matrix: A matrix **X** for which $\mathbf{XX}'$ has at least one *eigenvalue* near zero, so that numerical problems arise in computing $(\mathbf{XX}')^{-1}$.

Imputation: A procedure for dealing with *missing values* in which each missing observation is estimated to 'complete' the data set. The mean of a variable calculated from the available data on a variable might, for example, be used to replace the missing values of the variable. In practice, particularly for *multiple imputation* of missing values in *multivariate data*, far more complex estimation procedures involving *maximum likelihood estimation* are likely to be used. It must be remembered, however, that analysing 'filled in' data as if they were complete is likely to lead to overstatement of precision, i.e., standard errors that are underestimated, stated *P-values* that are too small and *confidence intervals* that do not cover the true parameter at the stated rate. See also **EM algorithm**.

Incidence: A measure of the rate at which people without a disease develop the disease during a specific period of time. Calculated as

$$\text{incidence} = \frac{\text{number of new cases of a disease over a period of time}}{\text{population at risk of the disease in the time period}}$$

it measures the appearance of disease. See also **prevalence**.

Incomplete block design: An *experimental design* in which not all treatments are represented in each *block*. See also **balanced incomplete block design**.

Incomplete contingency tables: *Contingency tables* containing *structural zeros*.

Incubation period: The time elapsing between the receipt of infection and the appearance of symptoms.

Independence: Essentially, two events are said to be independent if knowing the outcome of one tells us nothing about the other. More formally, the concept is defined in terms of the probabilities of the two events. In particular, two events A and B are said to be independent if

$$P(A \text{ and } B) = P(A) \times P(B)$$

where $P(A)$ and $P(B)$ represent the probabilities of A and B. See also **conditional probability** and **Bayes' theorem**.

Independent samples t-test: See **Student's t-test**.

Independent variables: See **explanatory variables**.

Index of clumping: An index used primarily in the analysis of *spatial data*, to investigate the pattern of the population under study. The index is calculated from the counts, $x_1, x_2, \cdots, x_n$, obtained from *quadrant sampling* as

$$\text{ICS} = s^2/\bar{x} - 1$$

where $\bar{x}$ and s^2 are the mean and variance of the observed counts. If the population is 'clustered', the index will be large, whereas if the individuals are regularly spaced the index will be negative. The *sampling distribution* of ICS is unknown, even for simple models of the underlying mechanism generating the population pattern.

Index of dispersion: A statistic most commonly used in assessing whether or not a *random variable* has a *Poisson distribution*. For a set of observations, $x_1, x_2, \cdots, x_n$, the index is given by

$$D = \sum_{i=1}^{n} (x_i - \bar{x})^2 / \bar{x}$$

If the population distribution is Poisson, then D has approximately a *chi-squared distribution* with $n - 1$ degrees of freedom. See also **binomial index of dispersion**.

Index plot: A plot of some diagnostic quantity, for example, *Cook's distances*, obtained after the fitting of some model, against the corresponding observation number. Particularly suited to the detection of *outliers*.

Indicator variable: A term generally used for a *manifest variable* that is thought to be related to an underlying *latent variable* in the context of *structural equation models*.

Indirect standardization: The process of adjusting a crude mortality or morbidity rate for one or more variables by using a known *reference population*. It might, for example, be required to compare cancer mortality rates of single and married women, with adjustment being made for the likely different age distributions in the two groups. *Age-specific mortality rates* in the reference population are applied separately to the age distributions of the two groups to obtain the expected number of deaths in each. These can then be combined with the observed number of deaths in the two groups to obtain comparable mortality rates.

Individual differences scaling (INDSCAL): A form of *multidimensional scaling* that allows for individual differences in the perception of the stimuli by deriving weights for each subject that can be used to stretch or shrink the dimensions of the recovered geometrical solution.

INDSCAL: Acronym for **individual differences scaling**.

Infant mortality rate: The ratio of the number of deaths during a calendar year among infants under one year of age to the total number of live births during that year. Often considered as a particularly responsive and sensitive index of the health status of a country or geographical area. The table below gives the rates per 1000 births in England, Wales, Scotland and Northern Ireland in both 1971 and 1992.

	1971	**1992**
England	17.5	6.5
Wales	18.4	5.9
Scotland	19.9	6.8
NI	22.7	6.0

Infectious period: A term used in describing the progress of an epidemic for the time following the *latent period* during which a patient infected with the disease is able to discharge infectious matter in some way, and possibly communicate the disease to other susceptibles.

Infectivity: The probability of infection, given exposure to an infectious agent under specified conditions.

Inference: The process of drawing conclusions about a population on the basis of measurements or observations made on a sample of individuals from the population.

Infertile worker effect: The observation that working women may be relatively infertile, since having children may keep women away from work. See also **healthy worker effect**.

Influence: A term used primarily in *regression analysis* to denote the effect of each observation on the estimated regression parameters. One useful index of the influence of each observation is provided by the diagonal elements of the *hat matrix*.

Influential observation: An observation that has a disproportionate *influence* on one or more aspects of the estimate of a parameter, in particular, a *regression coefficient*. This influence may be due to differences from other subjects on the explanatory variables, an extreme value for the response variable, or a combination of these. *Outliers*, for example, are often also influential observations.

Information theory: A branch of applied probability theory applicable to many communication and signal processing problems in engineering and biology. Information theorists devote their efforts to quantitative examination of the following three questions:

- what is information?
- what are the fundamental limitations on the accuracy with which information can be transmitted?
- what design methodologies and computational algorithms yield practical systems for communication and storing information that perform close to the fundamental limits mentioned previously?

Informative censoring: *Censored observations* that occur for reasons related to treatment, for example, when treatment is withdrawn as a result of a deterioration in the physical condition of a patient. This form of censoring makes most of the techniques for the analysis of *survival data*, for example, strictly invalid.

Informative missing values: See **missing values**.

Informative prior: A term used in the context of *Bayesian inference* to indicate a *prior distribution* that reflects empirical or theoretical information regarding the value of an unknown parameter.

Informed consent: The voluntary consent given by a patient to participate in, usually, a *clinical trial*, after being informed of its purpose, method of treatment, procedure for assignment to treatment, benefits and risks associated with participation, and required data collection procedures and schedule.

Initial data analysis: The first phase in the examination of a data set, which consists of a number of informal steps, including

- checking the quality of the data,
- calculating simple summary statistics and constructing appropriate graphs.

The general aim is to clarify the structure of the data, obtain a simple descriptive summary, and perhaps get ideas for a more sophisticated analysis.

Instantaneous death rate: Synonym for **hazard function**.

Instrumental variable: A variable corresponding to an explanatory variable, x_i, that is correlated with x_i but has no effect on the response variable except indirectly through x_i. Such variables are useful in deriving *unbiased* estimates of *regression coefficients* when the explanatory variables contain *measurement error*. See also **regression dilution**.

Intention-to-treat analysis: A procedure in which all patients *randomly allocated* to a treatment in a *clinical trial* are analysed together as representing that treatment, whether or not they completed, or even received it. Here the initial random allocation not only decides the allocated treatment, it decides there and then how the patient's data will be analysed, whether or not the patient actually receives the prescribed treatment. This method is adopted to prevent disturbances to the prognostic balance achieved by randomization and to prevent possible *bias* from using *compliance*, a factor often related to outcome, to determine the groups for comparison.

Interaction: A term applied when two (or more) explanatory variables do not act independently on a response variable. See also **additive effect**.

Intercept: The parameter in an equation derived from a *regression analysis* corresponding to the *expected value* of the response variable when all the *explanatory variables* are zero.

Interim analyses: Analyses made prior to the planned end of a *clinical trial*, usually with the aim of detecting treatment differences at an early stage and thus preventing as many patients as possible receiving an 'inferior' treatment. Such analyses are often problematical, particularly if carried out in a haphazard and unplanned fashion.

Interlaboratory trials: Studies conducted to determine the accuracy of methods of laboratory measurements. In such trials one or several samples of identical material are analysed by a sample of laboratories. The main sources of variability are

- the operator who performs the measurement,
- the equipment used,
- the environment in which the measurement takes place.

In general the *repeatability* and *reproducibilty* of the measures are used as parameters in describing accuracy. See also **round robin study**.

International classification of diseases: A categorization of disease determined by an internationally representative group of experts who advise the World Health Organization. Each disease category is given a three digit code number, and almost all categories are further subdivided into subcategories with four digit numbers.

Interpolation: The process of determining a value of a function between two known values without using the equation of the function itself.

Interquartile range: A measure of spread given by the difference between the first and third *quartiles* of a sample.

Interrupted time series design: A study in which a single group of subjects is measured several times before and after some event or manipulation. Often also used to describe investigations of a single subject. See also **longitudinal data** and **N of 1 clinical trials**.

Interval censored observations: Observations that often arise in the context of studies of time elapsed to a particular event when subjects are not monitored continuously. Instead, the prior occurrence of the event of interest is detectable only at specific times of observation, for example, at the time of medical examination.

Interval estimate: See **estimate**.

Interval estimation: See **estimation**.

Interval variable: Synonym for **continuous variable**.

Intervened Poisson distribution: A *probability distribution* that can be used as a model for a disease in situations where the *incidence* is altered in the middle of a data collection period, due to preventative treatments taken by health service agencies. The mathematical form of the distribution is

$$P(\text{number of cases} = x) = [e^{\theta\rho}(e^{\theta} - 1)]^{-1}[(1+\rho)^x - \rho^x]\theta^x/x!$$

where $x = 1, 2, \cdots$. The parameters $\theta(> 0)$ and $\rho(0 \leq \rho \leq \infty)$ measure incidence and intervention respectively. A zero value of ρ is indicative of completely successful preventive treatments, whereas $\rho = 1$ is interpreted as a status quo in the incidence rate even after the preventive treatments are applied.

Intervention study: Synonym for **clinical trial.**

Interviewer bias: The *bias* that occurs in surveys of human populations because of the direct result of the action of the interviewer. This bias can arise for a variety of reasons, including failure to contact the right persons and systematic errors in recording the answers received from the respondent.

Intraclass contingency table: A table obtained from a *square contingency table* by pooling the frequencies of cells corresponding to the same pair of categories. Such tables arise frequently in genetics when the genotypic distribution at a single locus with r *alleles*, $A_1, A_2, \cdots, A_r$, is observed. Since A_iA_j is indistinguishable from A_jA_i, $i \neq j$, only the total frequency of the unordered pair A_iA_j is observed. Thus the data consist of the frequencies of homozygotes and the combined frequencies of heterozygotes.

Intraclass correlation: Although originally introduced in genetics to judge sib-ship correlations, the term is now most often used for the proportion of variance of an observation due to between subject variability in the 'true' scores of a measuring instrument. Specifically, if an observed value, x, is considered to be true score (t) plus measurement error (e), i.e.,

$$x = t + e$$

the intraclass correlation is

$$\frac{\sigma_t^2}{(\sigma_t^2 + \sigma_e^2)}$$

where σ_t^2 is the variance of t and σ_e^2 the variance of e. The correlation can be estimated from a study involving a number of raters giving scores to a number of patients.

Intrinsically non-linear models: See **non-linear models**.

Intrinsic error: A term most often used in a clinical laboratory to describe the variability in results caused by the innate imprecision of each analytical step.

Invariance: A property of a set of variables or a statistic that is left unchanged by a transformation. The variance of a set of observations is, for example, invariant under *linear transformations* of the data.

Inverse normal distribution: A *probability distribution* having the form

$$f(x) = \left(\frac{\lambda}{2\pi x^3}\right)^{\frac{1}{2}} \exp - \left\{\frac{\lambda(x-\mu)^2}{2\mu^2 x}\right\}, \quad x > 0$$

where μ and λ are both positive. A member of the *exponential family* which is skewed to the right.

Inverse polynomial functions: Functions useful for modelling many *dose–response* relationships in biology. For a particular dose or stimulus, x, the *expected value* of the response variable, y, is defined by

$$E(y) = \frac{x+\alpha}{\sum_{i=0}^{d} \beta_i (x+\alpha)^i}, \quad x \geq 0$$

The parameters, $\beta_1, \beta_2, \cdots, \beta_d$, define the shape of the dose–response curve, and α defines its position on the x axis. A particularly useful form of the function is obtained by setting $\alpha = 0$ and $d = 1$. The resulting curve is

$$E(y) = \frac{x}{\beta_0 + \beta_1 x}, \quad x \geq 0$$

which can be rewritten as

$$E(y) = \frac{k_1 x}{k_2 + x}$$

where $k_1 = 1/\beta_1$ and $k_2 = \beta_0/\beta_1$. This final equation is equivalent to the *Michaelis–Menten* equation.

Isobole: See **isobologram.**

Isobologram: A diagram used to characterize the *interactions* among jointly administered drugs or chemicals. The contour of constant response (i.e., the *isobole*), is compared with the 'line of additivity', i.e., the line connecting the single drug doses that yield the level of response associated with that contour. The interaction is described as *synergistic*, additive, or *antagonistic* according to whether the isobol is below, coincident with, or above the line of additivity. (See Fig. 37 opposite.)

Item difficulty: See **Rasch model**.

Item non-response: A term used about data collected in a survey to indicate that particular questions in the survey attract refusals, or responses that

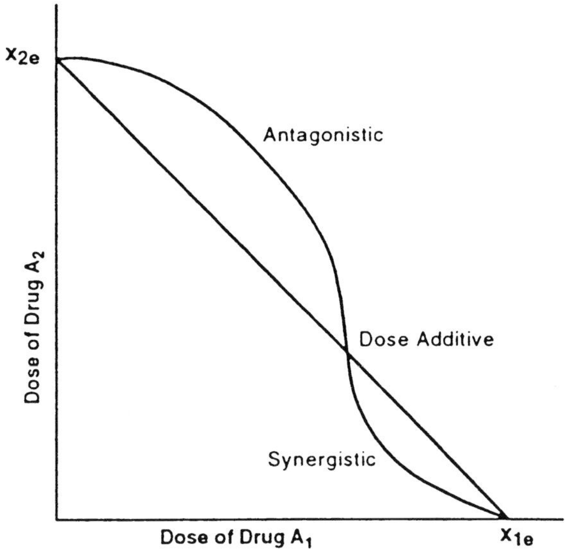

Fig 37 Isobologram.

cannot be coded. Often this type of *missing data* makes reporting of the overall response rate for the survey less relevant. See also **non-response**.

Item-response theory: The theory that states that a person's performance on a specific test item is determined by the amount of some underlying trait that the person has.

Item-total correlation: A widely used method for checking the homogeneity of a scale made up of several items. It is simply the *Pearson's product moment correlation coefficient* of an individual item, with the scale total calculated from the remaining items. The usual rule of thumb is that an item should correlate with the total above 0.20. Items with lower correlation should be discarded.

Iterated bootstrap: A two stage procedure in which the samples from the original *bootstrap* population are themselves bootstrapped. The technique can give *confidence intervals* of more accurate coverage than simple bootstrapping.

Iteration: The successive repetition of a mathematical process, using the result of one stage as the input for the next. Examples of procedures which involve iteration are *iterative proportional fitting*, the *Newton–Raphson method* and the *EM algorithm*.

Iteratively weighted least squares (IWLS) : A *weighted least squares* procedure in which the weights are revised or re-estimated at each iteration. In many cases the result is equivalent to *maximum likelihood estimation.*

Iterative proportional fitting: A procedure for the *maximum likelihood estimation* of the *expected frequencies* in *log-linear models*, particularly for models where such estimates cannot be found directly from simple calculations using relevant *marginal totals.*

IWLS: Abbreviation for **iteratively weighted least squares**.

J

Jaccard's coefficient: A *similarity coefficient* for use with data consisting of a series of *binary variables* that is often used in *cluster analysis*. The coefficient is given by

$$s_{ij} = \frac{a}{a + b + c}$$

where a, b and c are three of the frequencies in the 2×2 cross-classification of the variable values for subjects i and j. The critical feature of this coefficient is that 'negative matches' are excluded. See also **matching coefficient**.

Jackknife: A procedure for reducing *bias* in estimation and providing approximate *confidence intervals* in cases where these are difficult to obtain in the usual way. The principle behind the method is to omit each sample member in turn from the data,, thereby generating n separate samples each of size $n - 1$. The parameter of interest, θ, can now be estimated from each of these subsamples, giving a series of estimates, $\hat{\theta}_1, \hat{\theta}_2, \cdots, \hat{\theta}_n$. The jackknife estimator of the parameter is now

$$\tilde{\theta} = n\hat{\theta} - (n - 1)\frac{\sum_{i=1}^{n} \hat{\theta}_i}{n}$$

where $\hat{\theta}$ is the usual estimator using the complete set of n observations. The jackknife estimator of the standard error of $\hat{\theta}$ is

$$\hat{\sigma}_J = \left[\frac{(n - 1)}{n}\sum_{i=1}^{n}(\hat{\theta}_i - \bar{\theta})^2\right]^{\frac{1}{2}}$$

where $\bar{\theta} = \frac{1}{n}\sum_{i=1}^{n} \hat{\theta}_i$. A frequently used application is in *discriminant analysis*, for the estimation of the proportion of individuals misclassified by the derived *classification rule*. Calculated on the sample from which this rule is derived, the misclassification rate estimate is known to be optimistic. A jackknifed estimate obtained from calculating the discriminant function n times on the original observations, each time with one of the values removed, is usually a far more realistic measure of the performance of the derived classification rule.

Jewell's estimator: An estimator of the *odds ratio* given by

$$\hat{\psi} = \frac{ad}{(b+1)(c+1)}$$

where a, b, c and d are the cell frequencies in the *two-by-two contingency table* of interest. See also **Haldane's estimator**.

Jittering: A procedure for clarifying *scatter diagrams* when there is a multiplicity of points at many of the plotting locations, by adding a small amount of random variation to the data before graphing.

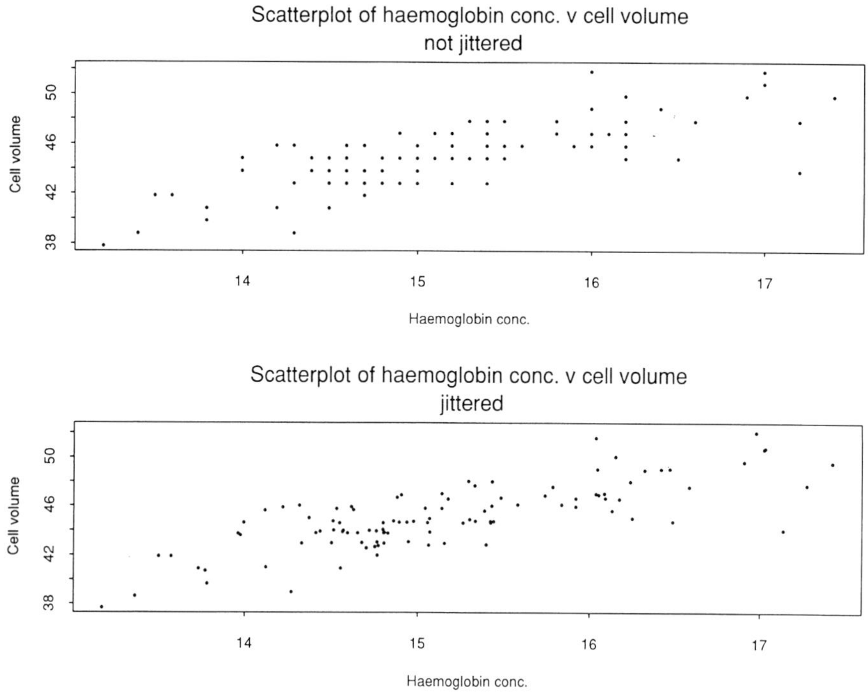

Fig 38 An example of 'jittering': first scatterplot shows raw data, second scatterplot shows data after being jittered.

Job-exposure matrix: A matrix, whose elements provide information on exposures to each of many industrial agents in each of many finely subdivided categories of occupation. A small example of such a matrix is given below;

Job-title	**Number in survey**	**Proportion exposed to**		
		S	**LO**	**CO**
Shoe factory workers	15	0.33	0.07	0.00
Stonemasons	6	0.00	0.00	0.00
Makers of metal moulds	22	0.18	0.36	0.64

S = Solvents: LO = Lubricating oils: CO = Cutting oils.

Joint distribution: Essentially synonymous with *multivariate distribution*, although used particularly as an alternative to *bivariate distribution* when two variables are involved.

Jonckheere's *k*-sample test: A *distribution-free method* for testing the equality of a set of location parameters against an *ordered alternative hypothesis*.

Jonckheere–Terpstra test: A test for detecting specific types of departures from independence in a *contingency table* in which both the row and column categories have a natural order. For example, suppose the *r* rows represent *r* distinct drug therapies at progressively increasing drug doses and the *c* columns represent *c* ordered responses. Interest in this case might centre on detecting a departure from independence, in which drugs administered at larger doses are more responsive than drugs administered at smaller ones. See also **linear-by-linear association test**.

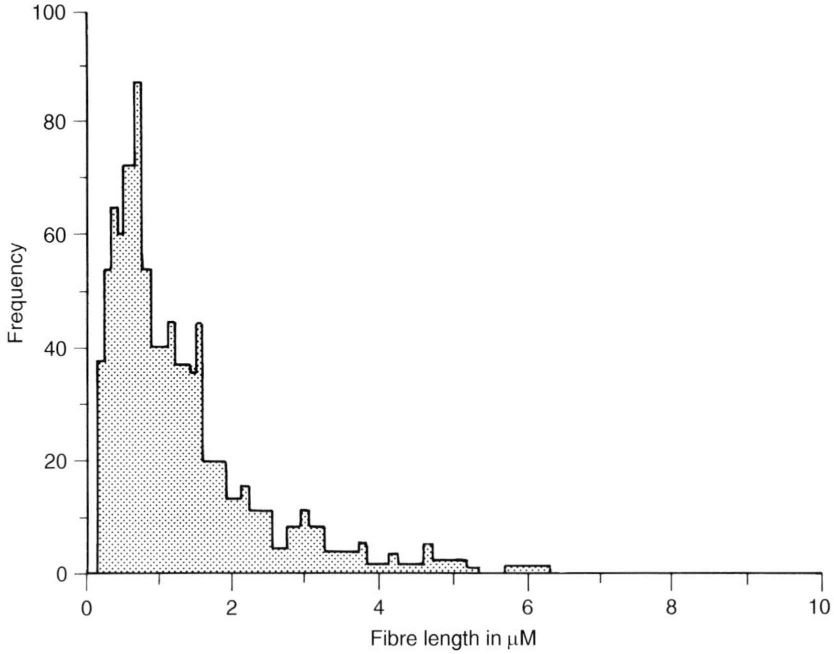

Fig 39 An example of a J-shaped distribution: the distribution of fibre size in air samples.

J-shaped distribution: An extremely *asymmetrical distribution* with its maximum frequency in the initial (or final) class and a declining or increasing frequency elsewhere.

Just identified model: See **identification**.

K

Kaiser's rule: A rule often used in *principal components analysis* for selecting the appropriate number of components. When the components are derived from the *correlation matrix* of the observed variables, the rule advocates retaining only those components with *eigenvalues* (variances) greater than unity. See also **scree plot**.

Kalman filter: A *recursive* procedure that provides an estimate of a signal when only the 'noisy signal' can be observed. Used as an estimation technique in the analysis of *time series* data.

Kaplan–Meier estimator: See **product limit estimator**.

Kappa coefficient: A chance corrected index of the agreement between, for example, judgements and diagnoses made by two raters. Calculated as the ratio of the observed excess over chance agreement to the maximum possible excess over chance, the coefficient takes the value unity when there is perfect agreement, and zero when observed agreement is equal to chance agreement.

Karnofsky rating scale: A measure of the ability to cope with everyday activities. The scale has eleven categories ranging from 0 (dead), to 10 (normal, no complaints, no evidence of disease). See also **Barthel index**.

Kendall's coefficient of concordance: Synonym for **coefficient of concordance**.

Kendall's tau statistics: Measures of the correlation between two sets of rankings. Kendall's tau (τ) itself is a *rank correlation coefficient* based on the number of inversions in one ranking as compared with another, i.e., on S, given by

$$S = P - Q$$

where P is the number of concordant pairs of observations, that is, pairs of observations such that their rankings on the two variables are in the same direction, and Q is the number of discordant pairs for which rankings on the two variables are in the reverse direction. The coefficient, τ, is calculated as

$$\tau = \frac{2S}{n(n-1)}$$

A number of other versions of τ have been developed that are suitable for measuring association in an $r \times c$ *contingency table* with both row and column variables having ordered categories. (Tau itself is not suitable since it assumes no tied observations). One example is the coefficient, τ_C, given by

$$\tau_C = \frac{2mS}{n^2(m-1)}$$

where $m = \min(r, c)$. See also **phi-coefficient, Cramer's V** and **contingency coefficient**.

Kermack and McKendrick's threshold theorem: A result concerned with the total size of an epidemic. It shows that the initial distribution of susceptibles is finally reduced to a point as far below some threshold value as it was originally above it.

Kernel estimators: See **kernel methods**.

Kernel function: See **kernel methods**.

Kernel methods: A generic term for methods of estimating a *probability distribution* using estimators of the form

$$\hat{f}(x) = \frac{1}{nh}\sum_{i=1}^{n} K\left(\frac{x - X_i}{h}\right)$$

where h is known as *window width* and K is the *kernel function*, which is such that

$$\int_{-\infty}^{\infty} K(u)\mathrm{d}u = 1$$

Essentially, such *kernel estimators* sum a series of 'bumps' placed at each of the observations. The kernel function determines the shape of the bumps, while h determines their width.

Kernel regression smoothing: A *distribution-free method* for smoothing data. In a single dimension, the method consists of the estimation of $m(x_i)$ in the relation

$$Y_i = m(x_i) + e_i$$

where $e_i, i = 1, \cdots, n$, are assumed to be symmetric errors with zero means. There are several methods for estimating the regression function, $m(x)$, for example, averaging the Y_i values that have x_i close to x.

K-means cluster analysis: A method of *cluster analysis* in which, from an initial partition of the observations into K clusters, each observation in turn is examined and reassigned, if appropriate, to a different cluster, in an attempt to optimize some predefined numerical criterion that measures, in some sense, the 'quality' of the cluster solution. Many such clustering criteria have been suggested, but the most commonly used arise from considering features of the *within groups, between groups* and *total matrices of sums of squares and cross products* $(\mathbf{W}, \mathbf{B}, \mathbf{T})$ that can be defined for every partition of the observations into a particular number of groups. The two most common of the clustering criteria arising from these matrices are

$$\text{minimization of trace}(\mathbf{W})$$
$$\text{minimization of determinant}(\mathbf{W})$$

The first of these has the tendency to produce 'spherical' clusters, the second to produce clusters that all have the same shape, although this will not necessarily be spherical. See also **agglomerative hierarchical clustering methods** and **divisive methods**.

Knots: See **spline functions**.

Knox's Tests: Tests designed to detect any tendency for patients with a particular disease to form a *disease cluster* in time and space. The tests are based on a *two-by-two contingency table*, formed from considering every pair of patients and classifying them as to whether the members of the pair were or were not closer than a critical distance apart in space, and as to whether the times at which they contracted the disease were closer than a chosen critical period.

Kolmogorov–Smirnov two sample method: A *distribution-free method* that tests for any difference between two population *probability distributions*. The test is based on the maximum absolute difference between the *cumulative distribution functions* of the samples from each population. *Critical values* are available in many statistical tables.

Kriging: A term used for the estimation or prediction of values in *spatial data*. For example, from the observed values, $y_1, y_2, \cdots, y_n$, of the concentration of a pollutant at n sites, $t_1, t_2, \cdots, t_n$, it may be required to estimate the concentration at a new nearby site, t_0.

Kronecker product of matrices: The result of multiplying the elements of an $m \times m$ matrix $\mathbf{A}$ term by term by those of an $n \times n$ matrix $\mathbf{B}$. The result is an $mn \times mn$ matrix. For example, if

$$\mathbf{A} = \begin{pmatrix} 1 & 2 \\ 3 & 4 \end{pmatrix} \text{ and } \mathbf{B} = \begin{pmatrix} 1 & 4 & 7 \\ 2 & 5 & 8 \\ 3 & 6 & 9 \end{pmatrix}, \text{then}$$

$$\mathbf{A} \bigotimes \mathbf{B} = \begin{pmatrix} 1 & 4 & 7 & 2 & 8 & 14 \\ 2 & 5 & 8 & 4 & 10 & 16 \\ 3 & 6 & 9 & 6 & 12 & 18 \\ 3 & 12 & 21 & 4 & 16 & 28 \\ 6 & 15 & 24 & 8 & 20 & 32 \\ 9 & 18 & 27 & 12 & 24 & 36 \end{pmatrix}$$

$\mathbf{A} \bigotimes \mathbf{B}$ is not in general equal to $\mathbf{B} \bigotimes \mathbf{A}$.

Kruskal–Wallis test: A *distribution-free method* that is the analogue of the *analysis of variance* of a *one-way design*. It tests whether the groups to be compared have the same population median. The *test statistic* is derived by ranking all the N observations from 1 to N regardless of which group they are in, and then calculating

$$H = \frac{12 \sum_{i=1}^{k} n_i (\bar{R}_i - \bar{R})^2}{N(N-1)}$$

where n_i is the number of observations in group i, $\bar{R}_i$ is the mean of their ranks, $\bar{R}$ is the average of all the ranks, given explicitly by $(N+1)/2$. When the *null hypothesis* is true, the test statistic has a *chi-squared distribution* with $k-1$ degrees of freedom.

Kurtosis: The extent to which the peak of a unimodal *probability distribution* or *frequency distribution* departs from the shape of a *normal distribution*, by either being more pointed (*leptokurtic*) or flatter (*platykurtic*). Usually measured for a probability distribution as

$$\mu_4 / \mu_2^2 - 3$$

where μ_4 is the fourth central *moment* of the distribution, and μ_2 is its variance. (Corresponding functions of the sample moments are used for frequency distributions). For a normal distribution, this index takes the value zero (other distributions with zero kurtosis are called *mesokurtic*), for one which is leptokurtic it is positive, and for a platykurtic curve it is negative.

L

Laboratory Information Management System (LIMS): A method for transferring laboratory generated data directly into a computer.

Lagrange multiplier test: Synonym for **score test**.

Large sample method: Any statistical method based on an approximation to a *normal distribution* or other *probability distribution* that becomes more accurate as sample size increases. See also **asymptotic distribution**.

Large simple trials (LST): *Clinical trials* in which exceptionally large numbers of patients with minimally restrictive entry criteria are used, and data collected only on essential *baseline characteristics* and outcomes.

Last observation carried forward (LOCF): A method for replacing the observations of patients who drop out of a *clinical trial* carried out over a period of time. It consists of substituting for each *missing value* the subject's last available assessment of the same type. Although widely applied, particularly in the pharmaceutical industry, its usefulness is very limited since it makes very unlikely assumptions about the data. See also **imputation**.

Latent class analysis: A method of assessing whether a set of observations involving *categorical variables*, in particular, *binary variables*, consists of a number of different groups or classes within which the variables are independent. Parameters in such models can be estimated by *maximum likelihood estimation* via the *EM algorithm*. Can be considered as either an analogue of *factor analysis* for categorical variables, or a model of *cluster analysis* for such data. See also **grade of membership model**.

Latent period: A term used, in describing an epidemic, for the time during which the disease develops purely internally within the infected person. See also **infectious period**.

Latent roots: Synonym for **eigenvalues**.

Latent variable: A variable that cannot be measured directly, but is assumed to be related to a number of observable or *manifest variables*. Examples include racial prejudice and social class. See also **indicator variable**.

Latent vectors: Synonym for **eigenvectors**.

Latin square: An experimental design aimed at removing from the experimental error the variation from two extraneous sources, so that a more sensitive test of the treatment effect can be achieved. The rows and columns of the square represent the levels of the two extraneous factors. The treatments are represented by roman letters arranged so that no letter appears more than once in each row and column. The following is an example of a 4×4 Latin square:

A	B	C	D
B	C	D	A
C	D	A	B
D	A	B	C

LD50: Abbreviation for **lethal dose 50**.

Lead time: The time gained in treating or controlling a disease when detection is earlier than usual, for example, in the presymptomatic stage. Such early detection is usually achieved through the use of a *screening study*.

Lead time bias: A term used, particularly with respect to cancer studies, for the bias that arises when the time from early detection to the time when the cancer would have been symptomatic is added to the *survival time* of each case.

Leaps-and-bounds algorithm: An *algorithm* used to find the optimal solution in problems that have a possibly very large number of solutions. Begins by splitting the possible solutions into a number of exclusive subsets, and limits the number of subsets that need to be examined in searching for the optimal solution by a number of different strategies. Often used in *all subsets regression* to restrict the number of models that have to be examined.

Least significant difference (LSD) test: An approach to comparing a set of means that controls the *familywise error rate* at some particular level, say α. The hypothesis of the equality of the means is tested first by an α-level *F-test*. If this test is not significant, then the procedure terminates without making detailed inferences on pairwise differences; otherwise each pairwise difference is tested by an α-level *Student's t-test*.

Least squares estimation: A method used for estimating parameters, particularly in *regression analysis*, by minimizing the difference between the observed response and the value predicted by the model. For example, if the *expected value* of a response variable y is of the form

$$E(y) = \alpha + \beta x$$

where x is an explanatory variable, then least squares estimators of the parameters α and β may be obtained from n pairs of sample values, $(x_1, y_1), (x_2, y_2), \cdots, (x_n, y_n)$, by minimizing S, given by

$$S = \sum_{i=1}^{n} (y_i - \alpha - \beta x_i)^2$$

to give

$$\hat{\alpha} = \bar{y} - \hat{\beta}\bar{x}$$

$$\hat{\beta} = \frac{\sum_{i=1}^{n}(x_i - \bar{x})(y_i - \bar{y})}{\sum_{i=1}^{n}(x_i - \bar{x})^2}$$

Often referred to as *ordinary least squares*, to differentiate this simple version of the technique from more involved versions, such as *weighted least squares* and *iteratively weighted least squares*. See also **Gauss-Markov theorem**.

Ledermann model: A model for the *probability distribution* of alcohol consumption in the population of drinkers. Empirical data appear to indicate that alcohol consumption has a *log-normal distribution*.

Length biased sampling: The *bias* that arises in a sampling scheme based on patient visits, when some individuals are more likely to be selected than others simply because they make more frequent visits. In a *screening study* for cancer, for example, the sample of cases detected is likely to contain an excess of slow-growing cancers compared to the sample diagnosed positive because of their symptoms.

Leptokurtic curve: See **kurtosis**.

Leslie matrix model: A model often applied in demographic and animal population studies, in which the vector of the number of individuals of each age at time t, $\mathbf{N}_t$, is related to the initial number of individuals of each age, $\mathbf{N}_0$, by the equation

$$\mathbf{N}_t = \mathbf{M}^t \mathbf{N}_0$$

where $\mathbf{M}$ is what is known as the *population projection matrix*, given by

$$\mathbf{M} = \begin{pmatrix} B_0 & B_1 & B_2 & \cdots & B_{v-1} & B_v \\ P_0 & 0 & 0 & \cdots & 0 & 0 \\ 0 & P_1 & 0 & \cdots & 0 & 0 \\ \vdots & \vdots & \vdots & \cdots & \vdots & \vdots \\ 0 & 0 & 0 & \cdots & P_{v-1} & P_v \end{pmatrix}$$

where B_x equals the number of females born to females of age x in one unit of time that survive to the next unit of time, P_x equals the proportion of females of age x at time t that survive to time $t+1$ and v is the greatest age attained.

Lethal dose 50 (LD50): The administered dose of a compound that causes death to 50% of the animals during a specified period, in an experiment involving toxic material.

Leverage points: A term used in *regression analysis* for those observations that have an extreme value on one or more explanatory variables. The effect of such points is to force the fitted model close to the observed value of the response, leading to a small *residual*. See also **hat matrix, influence** and **Cook's distance**.

Lexis diagram: A diagram for displaying the simultaneous effects of two time scales (usually age and calendar time) on a rate. For example, mortality rates from cancer of the cervix depend upon age, as a result of the age-dependence of the *incidence*, and upon calendar time as a result of changes in

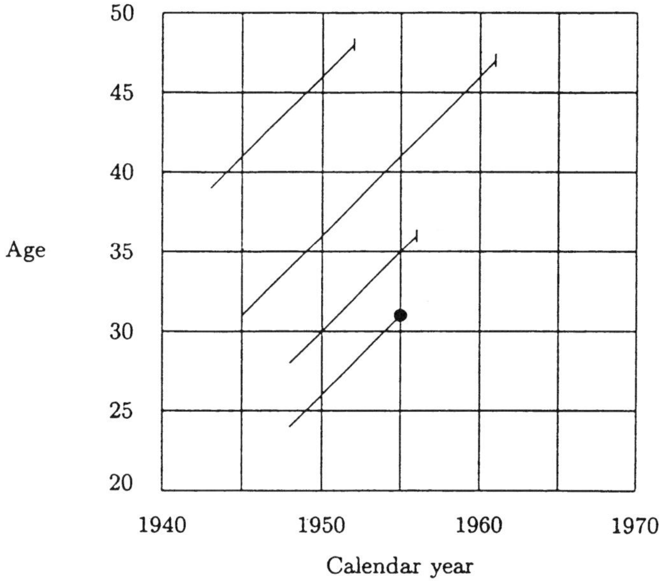

Fig 40 A Lexis diagram showing age and calender period.

treatment, population screening and so on. The main feature of such a diagram is a series of rectangular regions corresponding to a combination of two time bands, one from each scale. Rates for these combinations of bands can be estimated by allocating failures to the rectangles in which they occur, and dividing the total observation time for each subject between rectangles according to how long the subjects spend in each.

Lie factor: A quantity suggested by Tufte for judging the honesty of a graphical presentation of data. Calculated as

$$\frac{\text{apparent size of effect shown in graph}}{\text{actual size of effect in data}}$$

Values close to unity are desirable, but it is not uncommon to find values close to zero and greater than five. The example shown has a lie factor of about 2.8. (See Fig. 41 opposite.)

Life expectancy: The expected number of years remaining to be lived by persons of a particular age. For example, according to the US life table for 1979–1981, the life expectancy at birth is 73.88 years and that at age 40 is 36.79 years. The life expectancy of a population is a general indication of the capability of prolonging life. It is used to identify trends and to compare longevity.

Life table: A procedure used to compute chances of survival and death and remaining years of life, for specific years of age. An example of part of such a table is as follows:

Life table for white females, United States, 1949–1951

1	2	3	4	5	6	7
0	23.55	100 000	2355	97 965	7 203 179	72.03
1	1.89	97 465	185	97 552	7 105 214	72.77
2	1.12	97 460	109	97 406	7007 662	71.90
3	0.87	97 351	85	97 308	6 910 256	70.98
4	0.69	92 266	67	97 233	6 812 948	70.04
⋮	⋮	⋮	⋮	⋮	⋮	⋮
100	388.39	294	114	237	566	1.92

1 = year of age,
2 = death rate per 1000,
3 = number surviving of 100 000 born alive,
4 = number dying of 100 000 born alive,
5 = number of years lived by cohort,
6 = total number of years lived by cohort until all have died,
7 = average future years of life.

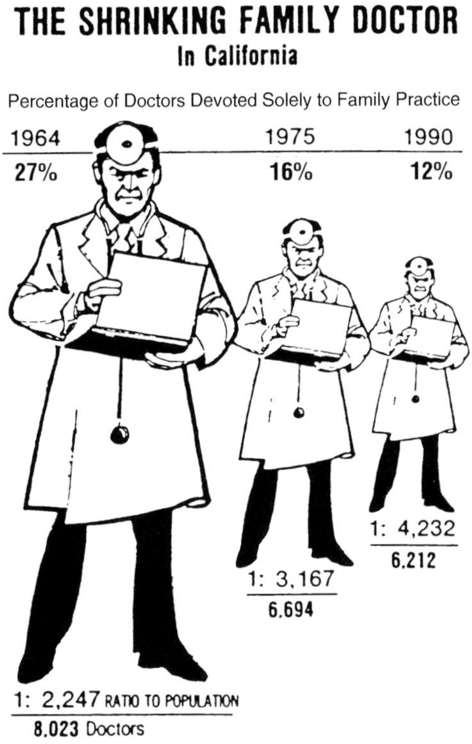
THE SHRINKING FAMILY DOCTOR
In California
Percentage of Doctors Devoted Solely to Family Practice
1964
27%
1975
16%
1990
12%
1: 2,247 RATIO TO POPULATION
8,023 Doctors
1: 3,167
6,694
1: 4,232
6,212

Fig 41 A diagram with a lie factor of about 2.8.

Life table analysis: A procedure often applied in *prospective studies* to examine the distribution of mortality and/or morbidity in one or more diseases in a *cohort study* of patients over a fixed period of time. For each specific increment in the follow-up period, the number entering the period, the number leaving during the period, and the number either dying from the disease (mortality) or developing the disease (morbidity), are all calculated. It is assumed that an individual not completing the follow-up period is exposed for half this period, thus enabling the data for those 'leaving' and those 'staying' to be combined into an appropriate denominator for the estimation of the percentage dying from or developing the disease. The advantage of this approach is that all patients, not only those who have been involved for an extended period, can be included in the estimation process.

Lifetime tumour rate: A term most often encountered in animal research, and defined as the probability that an animal dies with a tumour sometime during its lifetime, or, during an experiment with a terminal sacrifice, at some particular time point.

Likelihood: The probability of a set of observations, given the value of some parameter or set of parameters. For example, the likelihood of a *random sample* of n observations, $x_1, x_2, \cdots, x_n$, with *probability distribution*, $f(x, \theta)$, is given by

$$L = \prod_{i=1}^{n} f(x_i, \theta)$$

This function is the basis of *maximum likelihood estimation*. In many applications, the likelihood involves several parameters, only a few of which are of interest to the investigator. The remaining *nuisance parameters* are necessary in order that the model make sense physically, but their values are largely irrelevant to the investigation and the conclusions to be drawn. Since there are difficulties in dealing with likelihoods that depend on a large number of incidental parameters (for example, maximizing the likelihood will be more difficult) some form of modified likelihood is sought which contains as few of the uninteresting parameters as possible. A number of possibilities are available. For example, the *marginal likelihood* (often also called the *restricted likelihood*) eliminates the nuisance parameters by transforming the original variables in some way, or by working with some form of marginal variable. The *profile likelihood*, with respect to the parameters of interest, is the original likelihood, partially maximized with respect to the nuisance parameters. See also **quasi-likelihood** and **likelihood ratio**.

Likelihood distance test: A procedure for the detection of *outliers* that uses the difference between the *log-likelihood* of the complete data set and the log-likelihood when a particular observation is removed. If the difference is large, then the observation involved is considered an outlier.

Likelihood ratio: The ratio of the *likelihoods* of the data under two hypotheses, H_0 and H_1. Can be used to assess H_0 against H_1 since, under H_0, the statistic, λ, given by

$$\lambda = -2 \ln \frac{L_{H_0}}{L_{H_1}}$$

has approximately a *chi-squared distribution* with degrees of freedom equal to the difference in the number of parameters in the two hypotheses. See also $\mathbf{G^2}$, **deviance, goodness-of-fit statistics** and **Bartlett's adjustment factor**.

Likert scales: Scales often used in studies of attitudes, in which the raw scores are based on graded alternative responses to each of a series of questions. For example, the subject may be asked to indicate his/her degree of agreement with each of a series of statements relevant to the attitude. A number is attached to each possible response, e.g., 1: strongly approve; 2: approve; 3: undecided; 4: disapprove; 5: strongly disapprove; and the sum of these used as the composite score. A commonly used Likert-type scale in medicine is the *Apgar score* used to appraise the status of newborn infants. This is the sum of the points (0, 1 or 2) allotted for each of five items:

- heart rate (over 100 beats per minute, 2 points; slower, 1 point; no beat, 0 points);
- respiratory effort;
- muscle tone;
- response to stimulation by a catheter in the nostril;
- skin colour.

LIMS: Abbreviation for **Laboratory Information Management System**.

Linear-by-linear association test: A test for detecting specific types of departure from independence in a *contingency table* in which both the row and column categories have a natural order. See also **Jonckheere–Terpstra test**.

Linear estimator: An estimator which is a *linear function* of the observations, or of sample statistics calculated from the observations.

Linear function: A function of a set of variables, parameters, etc., that does not contain powers or cross-products of the quantities. For example, the following are all such functions of three variables, x_1, x_2 and x_3:

$$y = x_1 + 2x_2 + x_3$$
$$z = 6x_1 - x_3$$
$$w = 0.34x_1 - 2.4x_2 + 12x_3$$

Linearizing: The conversion of a *non-linear model* into one that is linear, for the purpose of simplifying the estimation of parameters. A common example of the use of the procedure is in association with the *Michaelis–Menten equation*

$$B = \frac{B_{\max} F}{K_{\mathrm{D}} + F}$$

where B and F are the concentrations of bound and free ligand at equilibrium, and the two parameters, $B_{\max}$ and K_{D} are known as capacity and affinity. This equation can be reduced to a linear form in a number of ways, for example:

$$\frac{1}{B} = \frac{1}{B_{\max}} + \frac{K_{\mathrm{D}}}{B_{\max}} \left(\frac{1}{F}\right)$$

is linear in terms of the variables $\frac{1}{B}$ and $\frac{1}{F}$. The resulting linear equation is known as the *Lineweaver–Burk equation*.

Linear logistic regression: Synonym for **logistic regression**.

Linear model: A model in which the *expected value* of a *random variable* is expressed as a *linear function* of the parameters in the model. Examples of linear models are

$$E(y) = \alpha + \beta x$$
$$E(y) = \alpha + \beta x + \gamma x^2$$

where x and y represent variable values and α, β and γ parameters. Note that the linearity applies to the parameters not to the variables. See also **linear regression** and **generalized linear models**.

Linear regression: A term usually reserved for the simple *linear model* involving a response, y, that is a *continuous variable* and a single explanatory variable, x, related by the equation

$$E(y) = \alpha + \beta x$$

where E denotes the *expected value*. See also **multiple regression** and **least squares estimation**.

Linear transformation: A transformation of q variables, $x_1, x_2, \cdots, x_q$, given by the q equations

$$\begin{aligned} y_1 &= a_{11}x_1 + a_{12}x_2 + \cdots + a_{1q}x_q \\ y_2 &= a_{21}x_1 + a_{22}x_2 + \cdots + a_{2q}x_q \\ &\vdots \\ y_q &= a_{q1}x_1 + a_{q2}x_2 + \cdots + a_{qq}x_q \end{aligned}$$

Such a transformation is the basis of *principal components analysis*.

Linear trend: A relationship between two variables in which the values of one change at a constant rate as the other increases.

Lineweaver–Burk equation: See **linearizing**.

Link function: See **generalized linear model**.

Linkage analysis: A method used for testing the hypothesis that a genetic marker of known location is on a different chromosome from a gene postulated to govern susceptibility to a disease.

Linkage map: A chromosome map showing the relevant positions of the known genes in the chromosomes of a given species.

LISREL: A computer program for fitting *structural equation models* involving *latent variables*. See also **EQS**.

Literature controls: Patients with the disease of interest who have received, in the past, one of two treatments under investigation, and for whom results have been published in the literature, now used as a control group for patients currently receiving the alternative treatment. Such a control group clearly requires careful checking for comparability. See also **historical controls**.

Loading matrix: See **factor analysis**.

Locally weighted regression: A method of *regression analysis* in which polynomials of degree one (linear) or two (quadratic) are used to approximate the regression function in particular 'neighbourhoods' of the space of the explanatory variables. Often useful for *smoothing scatter diagrams*, to allow any structure to be seen more clearly, and for identifying possible non-linear relationships between the response and explanatory variables. A *robust estimation* procedure (usually known as *lowess*) is used to guard against deviant points distorting the smoothed points. Essentially, the process involves an adaptation of *iteratively weighted least squares*. The example shown illustrates a situation in which the locally weighted regression differs considerably from the *linear regression* of y on x as fitted by *least squares estimation*.

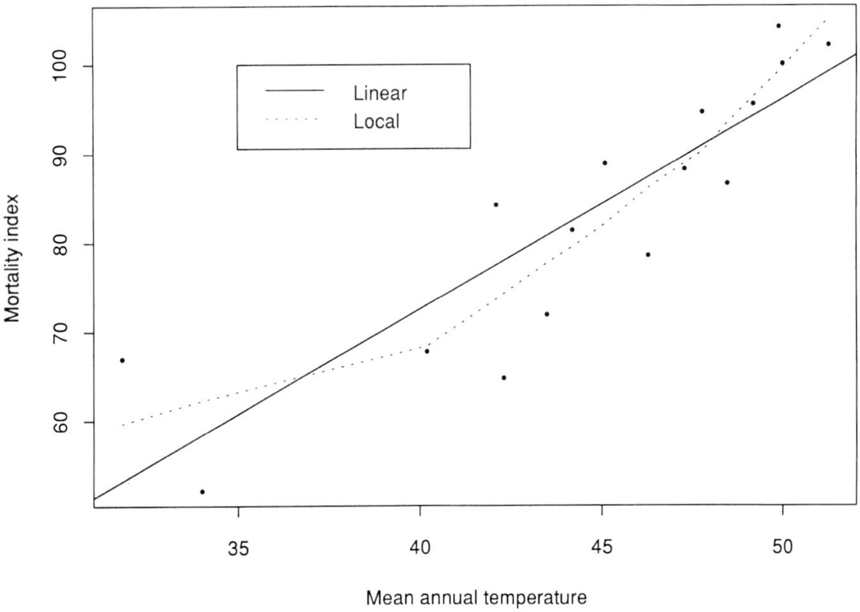

Fig 42 Scatterplot of breast cancer mortality rate versus temperature of region, with lines fitted by least squares estimation and by locally weighted regression.

Local odds ratio: The *odds ratio* of the *two-by-two contingency tables* formed from adjacent rows and columns in a larger *contingency table*.

Location: The notion of central or 'typical value' in a sample distribution. See also **mean, median** and **mode**.

LOCF: Abbreviation for **last observation carried forward**.

Lods: A term often used in *epidemiology* for the logarithm of an *odds ratio*. Also used in genetics for the logarithm of a *likelihood ratio*.

Logarithmic transformation: The transformation of a variable, x, obtained by taking $y = \ln(x)$. Often used when the *frequency distribution* of the variable, x, shows a moderate to large degree of *skewness*, in order to achieve normality.

Log-cumulative hazard plot: A plot used in *survival analysis* to assess whether particular parametric models for the *survival times* are tenable. Values of $\ln(-\ln \hat{S}(t))$ are plotted against $\ln t$, where $\hat{S}(t)$ is the estimated *survival function*. For example, an approximately linear plot suggests that the survival times have a *Weibull distribution*, and the plot can be used to provide rough estimates of its two parameters. When the slope of the line is close to unity, then an *exponential distribution* is implied.

Logistic growth model: The model appropriate for a *growth curve* when the rate of growth is proportional to the product of the size at the time and the amount of growth remaining. Specifically, the model is defined by the equation

$$y = \frac{\alpha}{1 + \gamma e^{-\beta t}}$$

where α, β and γ are parameters.

Logistic regression: A form of *regression analysis* used when the response variable is a *binary variable*. The method is based on the *logistic transformation* or *logit* of a proportion, namely

$$\text{logit}(p) = \ln \frac{p}{1-p}$$

As p tends to 0, logit(p) tends to $-\infty$, and as p tends to 1, logit(p) tends to ∞. The function logit(p) is a *sigmoid curve* that is symmetric about $p = 0.5$. Applying this transformation, this form of regression is written as

$$\ln \frac{p}{1-p} = \beta_0 + \beta_1 x_1 + \cdots + \beta_q x_q$$

where p = Prob(dependent variable = 1), and $x_1, x_2, \cdots, x_q$, are the explanatory variables. Using the logistic transformation in this way overcomes problems that might arise if p was modelled directly as a *linear function* of the explanatory variables, in particular, it avoids fitted probabilities outside the range (0,1). The parameters in the model can be estimated by *maximum likelihood estimation*. See also **conditional logistic regression**.

Logistic transformation: See **logistic regression**.

Logit: See **logistic regression**.

Logit confidence limits: The upper and lower ends of the *confidence interval* for the logarithm of the *odds ratio*, given by

$$\ln \hat{\psi} \pm z_{\alpha/2}\sqrt{\text{var}(\ln \hat{\psi})}$$

where $\hat{\psi}$ is the estimated odds ratio, $z_{\alpha/2}$ the *normal equivalent deviate* corresponding to a value of $\frac{\alpha}{2}$, $(1-\alpha)$ being the chosen size of the confidence interval. The variance term may be estimated by

$$\hat{\text{var}}(\ln \hat{\psi}) = \frac{1}{a} + \frac{1}{b} + \frac{1}{c} + \frac{1}{d}$$

where a, b, c and d are the frequencies in the *two-by-two contingency table* from which $\hat{\psi}$ is calculated. The two limits may be exponentiated to yield a corresponding confidence interval for the odds ratio itself.

Log-likelihood: The logarithm of the *likelihood*. Generally easier to work with than the likelihood itself when using *maximum likelihood estimation*.

Log-linear models: Models for *count data* in which the logarithm of the *expected value* of a count variable is modelled as a *linear function* of parameters; the latter represent associations between pairs of variables and higher order interactions between more than two variables. Estimated expected frequencies under particular models are found from *iterative proportional fitting*. Such models are, essentially, the equivalent, for frequency data, of the models for continuous data used in *analysis of variance*, except that interest usually now centres on parameters representing interactions, rather than those for main effects. See also **generalized linear model**.

Lognormal distribution: The *probability distribution* of a variable, x, for which $\ln(x-a)$ has a *normal distribution* with mean μ and variance σ^2. The specific form of the distribution is

$$f(x) = \frac{1}{\sigma(x-a)\sqrt{2\pi}}\exp\left[-\frac{1}{2\sigma^2}\left\{\ln\left(\frac{x-a}{\sigma}\right)^2\right\}\right]$$

Logrank test: A method for comparing the *survival times* of two or more groups of subjects, that involves the calculation of observed and *expected frequen-*

cies of failures in separate time intervals. The relevant *test statistic* is, essentially, a comparison of the observed number of deaths occurring at each particular time point with the number to be expected if the survival experience of the two groups is the same.

LOGXACT: A specialized statistical package that provides exact inference capabilities for *logistic regression*.

Longini–Koopman model: In *epidemiology*, a model for primary and secondary infection, based on the characterization of the *extra-binomial variation* in an infection rate that might arise due to the 'clustering' of the infected individuals within households. The assumptions underlying the model are:

- a person may become infected at most once during the course of the epidemic;
- all persons are members of a closed 'community'. In addition each person belongs to a single 'household'. A household may consist of one or several individuals;
- the sources of infection from the community are distributed homogeneously throughout the community. Household members mix at random within the household;
- each person can be infected either from within the household or from the community. The probability that a person is infected from the community is independent of the number of infected members in his or her household.

The probability that exactly k additional individuals will become infected for a household with s initial susceptibles and j initial infections is

$$P(k|s,j) = \binom{s}{k} P(k|k,j) B^{(s-k)} Q^{(j+k)(s-k)}, \quad k = 0, 1, \cdots, s-1$$

$$P(s|s,j) = 1 - \sum_{k=0}^{s-1} P(k|s,k)$$

where B is the probability that a susceptible individual is not infected from the community during the course of the infection, and Q is the probability that a susceptible person escapes infection from a single infected household member.

Longitudinal data: Data arising when each of a number of subjects or patients give rise to a vector of measurements representing the same variable observed at a number of different time points. Such data combine elements of *multivariate data* and *time series* data. They differ from the former, however, in that only a single variable is involved, and from the latter in consisting of a (possibly) large number of short series, one from each subject, rather than a single long series. Such data can be collected either prospectively, following subjects forward in time, or retrospectively, by extracting measurements on each person from historical records. This type of data is also often known as *repeated measures data*, particularly in the social and behavioural sciences, although in these disciplines such data are more likely to arise from observing individuals repeatedly under different experimental conditions, rather than from a simple time sequence. Special statistical methods are often needed for the analysis of this type of data because the set of measurements on one subject tend to be intercorrelated. This correlation must be taken into account to draw valid scientific inferences. See also **Greenhouse–Geisser correction, Huynh–Feldt correction, compound symmetry, generalized estimating equations, Mauchly test** and **split-plot design**.

Longitudinal studies: Studies that give rise to *longitudinal data*. The defining characteristic of such a study is that subjects are measured repeatedly through time.

Loss function: See **decision theory**.

Low-dose extrapolation: The process applied to the results from *bioassays* for carcinogenicity conducted in animals at doses that are generally well above human exposure levels, in order to assess risk in humans.

Lower triangular matrix: A matrix in which all the elements above the main diagonal are zero. An example is the folowing,

$$\mathbf{L} = \begin{pmatrix} 1 & 0 & 0 & 0 \\ 2 & 3 & 0 & 0 \\ 1 & 1 & 3 & 0 \\ 1 & 5 & 6 & 7 \end{pmatrix}$$

Lowess: See **locally weighted regression**.

LSD: Abbreviation for **least significant difference**.

LST: Abbreviation for **large simple trial**.

L-statistics: *Linear functions* of *order statistics* often used in estimation problems because they are typically computationally simple.

Lung cancer model: A proposed model for the relationship between smoking and lung cancer, given by

$$I_x = bNK(x - w)^{K-1}$$

where I_x is the *age-specific death rate* at age x, N is the number of cigarettes smoked per week, w is the age of starting smoking and K is a constant. The difference $x - w$ gives the period of exposure to tobacco smoke. The value of K has been determined empirically to be about 8.5.

Lung ventilation/perfusion ratio: The ratio of air flow to blood flow in the lung, usually denoted by V_A/Q. A small value of the ratio corresponds to a portion of the lung where the air flow is severely restricted, while a large value corresponds to a part of the lung with little blood flow. The example shown is for a healthy well-perfused, well-ventilated lung.

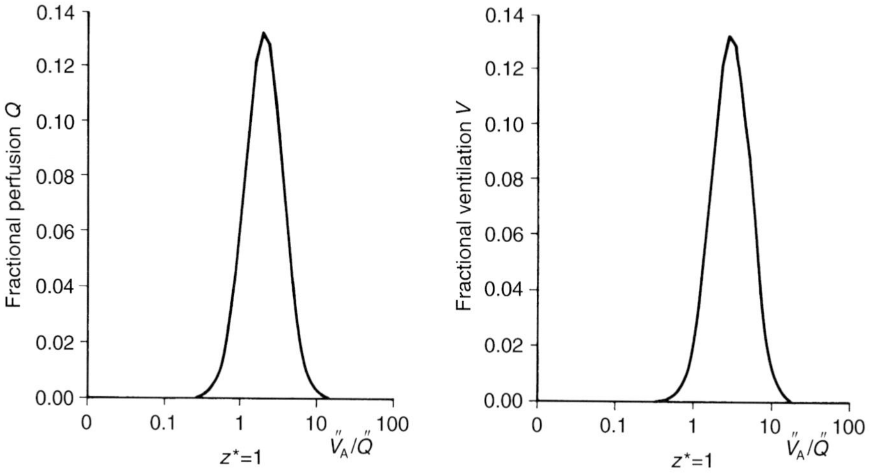

Fig 43 Lung ventilation/perfusion ratio diagram.

M

Mahalanobis D^2: A measure of the distance between two groups of individuals, given by

$$D^2 = (\bar{\mathbf{x}}_1 - \bar{\mathbf{x}}_2)'\mathbf{S}^{-1}(\bar{\mathbf{x}}_1 - \bar{\mathbf{x}}_2)$$

where $\bar{\mathbf{x}}_1$ and $\bar{\mathbf{x}}_2$ are the *mean vectors* of the two groups and $\mathbf{S}$ is a *weighted average* of the *variance–covariance matrices* of the two groups, $\mathbf{S}_1$ and $\mathbf{S}_2$, i.e.,

$$\mathbf{S} = \frac{n_1\mathbf{S}_1 + n_2\mathbf{S}_2}{n_1 + n_2}$$

where n_1 and n_2 are the sample sizes in the two groups. See also **Hotelling's T^2 test**.

Main effect: An estimate of the independent effect of (usually) a factor variable on a response variable in *analysis of variance*.

Mainframes: High speed general purpose computers with a very large storage capacity.

Majority rule: A requirement that the majority of a series of *diagnostic tests* are positive before declaring that a patient has a particular complaint. See also **unanimity rule**.

Mallow's C_k statistic: An index used in *regression analysis* as an aid in choosing the 'best' subset of *explanatory variables*. The index is defined as

$$C_k = \sum_{i=1}^{n} (y_i - \hat{y}_i^{(k)})^2/s^2 - n + 2q$$

where n is the number of observations, y_i is the observed value of the response variable for individual i, $\hat{y}_i^{(k)}$ is the corresponding predicted value from a model with a particular set of k explanatory variables, and s^2 is the *residual mean square* after regression on the complete set of q explanatory variables. The model chosen is the one with the minimum value of C_k. See also **Akaike's information criterion** and **all subsets regression**.

Manhattan distance: Synonym for **city-block distance**.

Manifest variable: A variable that can be measured directly, in contrast to a *latent variable.*

Mann–Whitney test: A *distribution-free method* used as an alternative to the *Student's t-test* for assessing whether two populations have the same location. Given a sample of observations from each population, all the observations are ranked as if they were from a single sample, and the *test statistic* is the sum of the ranks in the smaller group. Tables giving *critical values* of the test statistic are available, and for moderate and large sample sizes, a normal approximation can be used.

MANOVA: Acronym for **multivariate analysis of variance**.

Mantel–Haenszel estimator: An estimator of the assumed common *odds ratio* in a series of *two-by-two contingency* tables arising from different populations, for example, occupation, country of origin, etc. Specifically, the estimator is defined as

$$\omega = \sum_{i=1}^{k} a_i d_i / \sum_{i=1}^{k} c_i b_i$$

where k is the number of two-by-two tables involved and a_i, b_i, c_i, d_i are the four counts in the ith table.

Maple: A computer system for both mathematical computation and computer algebra.

Mapping disease: The process of displaying the geographical variability of disease on maps using different colours, shading, etc. The idea is not new, but the advent of computers and computer graphics has made the procedure far simpler to implement. See also **cartogram**.

Mardia's multivariate normality test: A test that a set of *multivariate data* arise from a *multivariate normal distribution* against departures due to *kurtosis.* The test is based on the following multivariate kurtosis measure

$$b_{2,q} = \frac{1}{n}\sum_{i=1}^{n}\{(\mathbf{x}_i - \bar{\mathbf{x}})'\mathbf{S}^{-1}(\mathbf{x}_i - \bar{\mathbf{x}})\}^2$$

where q is the number of variables, n is the sample size, $\mathbf{x}_i$ is the vector of observations for subject i, $\bar{\mathbf{x}}$ is the *mean vector* of the observations, and $\mathbf{S}$ is the sample *variance–covariance matrix.* For large samples, under the hypothesis that the data arise from a multivariate normal distribution, $b_{2,q}$ has a *normal distribution* with mean $q(q+2)$ and variance $8q(q+2)/n$.

Marginal homogeneity: A term applied to *square contingency tables* when the probabilities of falling in each category of the row classification equal the corresponding probabilities for the column classification. See also **Stuart–Maxwell test**.

Marginal likelihood: See **likelihood**.

Marginal matching: The *matching* of treatment groups in terms of means or other summary characteristics of the matching variables. Has been shown to be almost as efficient as the matching of individual subjects in some circumstances.

Marginal models: Synonym for **population averaged model**.

Marginal probability distribution: The *probability distribution* of a single variable, or combinations of variables, in a set of *multivariate data*. Obtained from the multivariate distribution by integrating over the other variables.

Marginal totals: A term often used for the total number of observations in each row and each column of a *contingency table*.

Markers of disease progression: Quantities that form a general *monotonic sequence* throughout the course of a disease and assist with its modelling. In general, such quantities are highly prognostic in predicting the future course. An example is CD4 cell count (cells per μL), which is generally accepted as the best marker of HIV disease progression.

Markov chain: A discrete *stochastic process* in which the probability that a system will be in a given state on the $(k+1)$th trial depends only on the state of the system on the kth trial. (Sometimes known more specifically as a *first order Markov chain*, to differentiate it from processes depending on more than the immediate previous state.)

Markov illness–death model: A model in which live individuals are classified as either having, or not having, a disease A, and then move between these possibilities and death as indicated in the diagram shown overleaf.

Markov inequality: See **Chebyshev's inequality**.

Markov process: A *stochastic process* with the property that its state at any time in the future is dependent only on its present state, and is unaffected by any additional knowledge of the past history of the system. See also **random walk**.

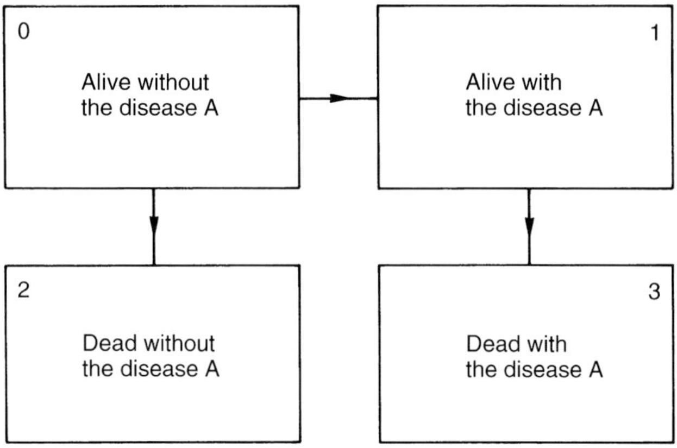

Fig 44 Markov illness–death model diagram.

Martingale: A *stochastic process*, or a sequence of *random variables*, which is such that the *expected value* of the $(n+1)$th random variable, conditional on the values of the first n, equals the value of the nth random variable.

Matchability: A term used most often in kidney transplantation for the probability that a patient will be offered a well-matched kidney from a random donor. Depends on the patient's tissue type, and also on the tissue type of other patients awaiting kidney transplantation.

Matched case–control study: See **retrospective study**.

Matched pairs: A term used for observations arising from either two individuals who are individually matched on a number of variables, for example, age, sex, or where two observations are taken on the same individual on two separate occasions. Essentially synonymous with **paired samples**.

Matched pairs *t*-test: A *Student's t-test* for the equality of the means of two populations, when the observations arise as *paired samples*. The test is based on the differences between the observations of the matched pairs. The *test statistic* is given by

$$t = \frac{\bar{d}}{s_d/\sqrt{n}}$$

where n is the sample size, $\bar{d}$ is the mean of the differences, and s_d their standard deviation. If the *null hypothesis* of the equality of the population means is true, then t has a *Student's t-distribution* with $n-1$ degrees of freedom.

Matched set: See **one:*m* matching**.

Matching: The process of making a study group and a comparison group comparable with respect to extraneous factors. Often used in *retrospective studies*, when selecting cases and controls, to control variation in a response variable due to sources other than those immediately under investigation. Several kinds of matching can be identified, the most common of which is when each case is individually matched with a control subject on the matching variables, such as age, sex, occupation. When the variable on which the matching takes place is continous, it is usually transformed into a series of categories (e.g., age), but a second method is to say that two values of the variable match if their difference lies between defined limits. This method is known as *caliper matching*. See also **paired samples**.

Matching coefficient: A *similarity coefficient* for data consisting of a number of *binary variables*, that is often used in *cluster analysis*. Given by

$$s_{ij} = \frac{a}{a+b+c+d}$$

where a, b, c and d are the four frequencies in the two-by-two cross-classification of the variable values for subjects i and j. See also **Jaccard's coefficient**.

Maternal mortality rate: A measure of the risk of dying from causes associated with child birth. Usually measured as

$$\text{maternal mortality rate} = \frac{\text{number of deaths from puerperal causes during a year}}{\text{number of live births in year}}$$

Matrix: A rectangular arrangement of numbers, algebraic functions, etc. Two examples are

$$\mathbf{A} = \begin{pmatrix} 1 & 1 & 2 \\ 2 & 1 & 7 \end{pmatrix}$$

$$\mathbf{B} = \begin{pmatrix} b_{11} & b_{12} \\ b_{21} & b_{22} \\ b_{31} & b_{32} \\ b_{41} & b_{42} \end{pmatrix}$$

Mauchly test: A test that a *variance–covariance matrix* of a set of *multivariate data* is a scalar multiple of the *identity matrix*, a property known as *sphericity*. Of most importance in the analysis of *longitudinal data*, where this property must hold for the *F-tests* in the *analysis of variance* of such data to be valid. See also **compound symmetry, Greenhouse–Geisser correction** and **Huynh–Feldt correction**.

Maximum F-ratio: Equivalent to *Hartley's test*. See also **Bartlett's test** and **Box's test**.

Maximum likelihood estimation (MLE): An estimation procedure involving maximization of the *likelihood* or the *log-likelihood* with respect to the parameters. Such estimators are particularly important because of their many desirable statistical properties, such as *consistency* and *asymptotic relative efficiency*. As an example, consider the number of successes, X, in a series of *random variables* from a *Bernoulli distribution* with success probability p. The likelihood is given by

$$P(X = x|p) = \binom{n}{x} p^x (1-p)^{n-x}$$

Differentiating the log-likelihood, L, with respect to p gives

$$\frac{\partial L}{\partial p} = \frac{x}{p} - \frac{n-x}{1-p}$$

Setting this equal to zero gives the estimator $\hat{p} = x/n$. See also **EM algorithm**.

Maximum tolerated dose: The highest possible dose of a drug that can be given with acceptable patient toxicity. This dose is usually determined in a *phase I clinical trial* and is the dose recommended for future studies. See also **Fibonacci dose escalation scheme**.

MCAR: Abbreviation for **missing completely at random**.

McNemar's test: A test for comparing proportions in data involving *paired samples*. The *test statistic* is given by

$$X^2 = \frac{(b-c)^2}{b+c}$$

where b is the number of pairs for which the individual receiving treatment A has a positive response and the individual receiving treatment B does not, and c is the number of pairs for which the reverse is the case. If the probability of a positive response is the same in each group, then X^2 has a *chi-squared distribution* with a single degree of freedom.

Mean: A measure of location or central value for a continuous variable. For a definition of the population value see *expected value*. For a sample of observations, $x_1, x_2, \cdots, x_n$, the measure is calculated as

$$\bar{x} = \frac{\sum_{i=1}^{n} x_i}{n}$$

Most useful when the data have a *symmetric distribution* and do not contain *outliers*. See also **median** and **mode**.

Mean–range plot: A graphical tool useful in selecting a transformation in *time series* analysis. The range is plotted against the mean for each seasonal period, and a suitable transformation chosen according to the appearance of the plot. If the range appears to be independent of the mean, for example, no transformation is needed. If the plot displays random scatter about a straight line then a logarithmic transformation is appropriate.

Mean square contingency coefficient: The square of the *phi-coefficient*.

Mean squared error: The *expected value* of the square of the difference between an estimator and the true value of a parameter. If the estimator is unbiased, then the mean squared error is simply the variance of the estimator. For a biased estimator the mean squared error is equal to the sum of the variance and the square of the *bias*.

Mean square ratio: The ratio of two *mean squares* in an *analysis of variance*.

Mean squares: The name used in the context of *analysis of variance* for estimators of particular variances of interest. For example, in the analysis of a *one way design*, the *within groups mean square* estimates the assumed common variance in the k groups (this is often also referred to as the *error mean square*).

Mean vector: A vector containing the mean values of each variable in a set of *multivariate data*.

Measurement error: Errors in reading, calculating or recording a numerical value. The difference between observed values of a variable recorded under similar conditions and some fixed true value.

Measures of association: Numerical indices quantifying the strength of the statistical dependence of two or more qualitative variables. See also **phi-coefficient** and **Goodman–Kruskal measures of association**.

Median: The value in a set of ranked observations that divides the data into two parts of equal size. When there is an odd number of observations the median is the middle value. When there is an even number of observations the median is calculated as the average of the two central values. Provides a measure of location of a sample that is suitable for *asymetric distributions* and is also relatively insensitive to the presence of *outliers*. See also **mean**, **mode**, **spatial median** and **bivariate Oja median**.

Mediancentre: Synonym for **spatial median**.

Median effective dose (ED50): A quantity used to characterise the potency of a stimulus. Given by the amount of the stimulus that produces a response in 50% of the cases to which it is applied.

Median lethal dose: Synonym for **lethal dose 50**.

Medical audit: The examination of data collected from routine medical practice with the aim of identifying areas where improvements in efficiency and/or quality might be possible.

MEDLINE: Medical Literature Analysis Retrieval System on line.

Mesokurtic curve: See **kurtosis**.

M-estimators: Robust estimators of parameters in statistical models that bound the *influence* of individual observations.

Meta-analysis: A collection of techniques whereby the results of two or more independent studies are statistically combined to yield an overall answer to a question of interest. The rationale behind this approach is to provide a test with more *power* than is provided by the separate studies themselves. The procedure has become increasingly popular in the last decade or so, but it is not without its critics, particularly because of the difficulties of knowing which studies should be included and to which population final results actually apply.

Method of moments: A procedure for estimating the parameters in a model by equating sample *moments* to their population values. A famous early example of the use of the procedure is in Pearson's description of estimating the five parameters in a *finite mixture distribution* with two univariate normal components. Little used in modern statistics, since the estimates are known to be less efficient than those given by alternative procedures such as *maximum likelihood estimation*.

Metric inequality: A property of some *dissimilarity coefficients*, such that the dissimilarity between two points i and j is less than or equal to the sum of their dissimilarities from a third point k. Specifically,

$$\delta_{ij} \leq \delta_{ik} + \delta_{jk}$$

Indices satisfying this inequality are referred to as *distance measures*.

Michaelis-Menten equation: See **linearizing** and **inverse polynomial functions**.

Michael's test: A test that a set of data arise from a *normal distribution*. If the ordered sample values are $x_{(1)}, x_{(2)}, \cdots, x_{(n)}$, the test statistic is

$$D_{SP} = \max_i |g(f_i) - g(p_i)|$$

where

$$f_i = \Phi\{(x_{(i)} - \bar{x})/s\}$$

$$g(y) = \frac{2}{\pi}\sin^{-1}(\sqrt{(y)})$$

$$p_i = (i - \frac{1}{2})/n$$

$\bar{x}$ is the sample mean,

$$s^2 = \frac{1}{n}\sum_{i=1}^{n}(x_{(i)} - \bar{x})^2$$

and

$$\Phi(w) = \int_{-\infty}^{w} \frac{1}{\sqrt{2\pi}} e^{-\frac{1}{2}u^2} \mathrm{d}u$$

Critical values of D_{SP} are available in some statistical tables.

Mid P-value: An alternative to the conventional *P-value* that is used, in particular, in some analyses of discrete data, for example, *Fisher's exact test* on *two-by-two contingency tables*. In the latter, if $x = a$ is the observed value of the frequency of interest, and this is larger than the value expected, then the mid P-value is defined as

$$\text{mid P-value} = \tfrac{1}{2}\text{Prob}(x = a) + \text{Prob}(x > a)$$

In this situation, the usual P-value would be defined as $\text{Prob}(x \geq a)$.

Mid-range: The mean of the smallest and largest values in a sample. Sometimes used as a rough estimate of the mean of a *symmetrical distribution*.

MIMIC model: Abbreviation for **multiple indicator multiple cause model**.

Minimax rule: A term most often encountered when deriving *classification rules* in *discriminant analysis*. It arises from attempting to find a rule that safeguards against doing very badly on one population, and so uses the criterion of minimizing the maximum probability of misclassification in deriving the rule.

Minimization: A method for allocating patients to treatments in *clinical trials* which is usually an acceptable alternative to *random allocation*. The procedure ensures balance between the groups to be compared on *prognostic variables*, by allocating with high probability the next patient to enter the trial to whatever treatment would minimize the overall imbalance between the groups on the prognostic variables, at that stage of the trial. See also **biased coin method** and **block randomization**.

Minimum chi-squared estimation: A method of estimation that finds estimates of the parameters of some model of interest by minimizing the *chi-squared statistic* for assessing differences between observed values and those predicted by the model.

Minimum spanning tree: See **tree**.

MINITAB: A general purpose statistical software package, specifically designed to be useful for teaching purposes.

Minkowski distance: A *distance measure*, $d_{\mathbf{xy}}$, for two observations $\mathbf{x}' = [x_1, x_2, \cdots, x_q]$ and $\mathbf{y}' = [y_1, y_2, \cdots, y_q]$ from a set of *multivariate data*, given by

$$d_{\mathbf{xy}} = \left[\sum_{i=1}^{q}(x_i - y_i)^r\right]^{\frac{1}{r}}$$

When $r = 2$ this reduces to *Euclidean distance*.

Minnesota multiphasic personality inventory (MMPI): An empirically based test of adult psychopathology, designed to assess the major symptoms and signs of social and personal maladjustment commonly indicative of disabling psychological dysfunction. The inventory is used by clinicians in hospitals to assist with diagnosis of mental disorders and the selection of an appropriate method of treatment.

Misinterpretation of P-values: A *P-value* is commonly interpreted in a variety of ways that are incorrect. Most common are that it is the probability of the null hypothesis, and that it is the probability of the data having arisen by chance. For the correct interpretation, see the entry for **P-value**.

Missing completely at random (MCAR): See **missing values**.

Missing values: Observations missing from a set of data for some reason. Such values cause most problems for *longitudinal studies*, where they occur for a variety of reasons, for example, because subjects drop out of the study completely, or do not appear for one or other of the scheduled visits, or because of equipment failure. Common causes of subjects prematurely ceasing to participate include recovery, lack of improvement, unwanted signs or symptoms that may be related to the investigational treatment, unpleasant study procedures and intercurrent health problems. Missing values greatly complicate many methods of analysis and simply dealing with those individuals for which the data are complete can be unsatisfactory in many situations. Different approaches may be necessary for the analysis of data containing missing values, depending on whether they are thought to be *missing completely at random* or *informative*. In the former case the missing values are independent of both the observed data and the data that would have been available had they not been missing, and in the latter they are dependent on these unavailable data. See also **last observation carried forward, attrition** and **imputation**.

Mis-specification: A term sometimes applied in situations where the wrong model has been assumed for a particular set of observations.

Mitscherlich curve: A curve which may be used to model a *hazard function* that increases or decreases with time in the short term and then becomes constant. Its formula is

$$h(t) = \theta - \beta e^{-\gamma t}$$

where all three parameters, θ, β and γ, are greater than zero.

Mixed data: Data containing a mixture of *continuous variables, ordinal variables* and *categorical variables.*

Mixed-effects logistic regression: A generalization of standard *logistic regression* in which the intercept terms, α_i, are allowed to vary between subjects according to some *probability distribution*, $f(\alpha)$. In essence, these terms are used to model the possible different *frailties* of the subjects. For a single covariate, x, the model is

$$\text{logit}(P(y_{ij}|\alpha_i, x_{ij})) = \alpha_i + \beta x_{ij}$$

where y_{ij} is the binary response variable for the jth measurement on subject i, and x_{ij} is the corresponding covariate value. Here β measures the change in the conditional logit of the probability of a response of unity with the covariate, x, for individuals in each of the underlying risk groups described by α_i. The *population averaged model* for y_{ij} derived from this model is

$$P(y_{ij} = 1|x_{ij}) = \int (1 + e^{-\alpha-\beta x_{ij}})^{-1} f(\alpha) \mathrm{d}\alpha$$

Mixed effects model: A model usually encountered in the analysis of *longitudinal data*, in which some of the parameters are considered to have *fixed effects* and some to have *random effects*. For example, in a *clinical trial* with two treatment groups in which the response variable is recorded on each subject at a number of visits, the treatments would usually be regarded as having fixed effects and the subjects random effects.

Mixture experiments: Experiments that consist of varying the proportions of two or more ingredients and studying the change that occurs in the measured response that is assumed to be functionally related to ingredient composition. The controllable variables are proportionate amounts of the mixture in which the proportions are by volume, weight or mole fraction.

MLE: Abbreviation for **maximum likelihood estimation**.

MMPI: Abbreviation for **Minnesota multiphasic personality inventory**.

Mode: The most frequently occurring value in a set of observations. Occasionally used as a measure of location. See also **mean** and **median**.

Model: A description of the assumed structure of a set of observations, that can range from a fairly imprecise verbal account to, more usually, a formalised mathematical expression of the process assumed to have generated the observed data. The purpose of such a description is to aid in understanding the data. See also **deterministic model, logistic regression, multiple regression, random model** and **generalized linear models**.

Model building: A procedure which attempts to find the simplest model for a sample of observations that provides an adequate fit to the data. See also **parsimony principle**.

Mojena's test: A test for the number of groups when applying *agglomerative hierarchical clustering methods*. In detail, the procedure is to select the number of groups corresponding to the first stage in the *dendrogram* satisfying

$$\alpha_{j+1} > \bar{\alpha} + ks_\alpha$$

where $\alpha_0, \alpha_1, \cdots, \alpha_{n-1}$ are the fusion levels corresponding to stages with $n, n-1, \cdots, 1$ clusters, and n is the sample size. The terms $\bar{\alpha}$ and s_α are, respectively, the mean and unbiased standard deviation of the α values, and k is a constant, with values in the range 2.75–3.50 usually being recommended.

Moments: Values used to characterize the *probability distributions* of *random variables*. The kth moment about the origin for a variable x is defined as

$$\mu_k' = E(x^k)$$

so that μ_1' is simply the mean and generally denoted by μ. The kth moment about the mean, μ_k, is defined as

$$\mu_k = E(x - \mu)^k$$

so that μ_2 is the variance. Moments of samples can be defined in an analogous way, for example,

$$m_k' = \frac{\sum_{i=1}^{n} x_i^k}{n}$$

where $x_1, x_2, \cdots, x_n$ are the observed values. See also **method of moments**.

Monotonic decreasing: See **monotonic sequence**.

Monotonic increasing: See **monotonic sequence**.

Monotonic regression: A procedure for obtaining the curve that best fits a set of points, subject to the constraint that it never decreases. A central component of *non-metric scaling*.

Monotonic sequence: A sequence of numerical values is said to be *monotonic increasing* if each value is greater than or equal to the previous one, and *monotonic decreasing* if each value is less than or equal to the previous one. See also **ranking**.

Monte Carlo methods: Methods for finding solutions to mathematical and statistical problems by *simulation*.

Moral graph: Synonym for **conditional independence graph**.

Moran's *I*: A statistic used in the analysis of *spatial data* to detect *autocorrelation*. If $x_1, x_2, \cdots, x_n$ represent data values at n locations in space, and $\mathbf{W}$ is a matrix with elements w_{ij} equal to unity if i and j are neighbours and zero otherwise ($w_{ii} = 0$), then the statistic is defined as

$$I = \frac{n}{\mathbf{1}'\mathbf{W}\mathbf{1}} \frac{\mathbf{z}'\mathbf{W}\mathbf{z}}{\mathbf{z}'\mathbf{z}}$$

where $z_i = x_i - \bar{x}$ and $\mathbf{1}$ is an n-dimensional vector of ones. The statistic is like an ordinary *Pearson's product moment correlation coefficient* but the cross-product terms are calculated only between neighbours. If there is no spatial autocorrelation then I will be close to zero. Clustering in the data will lead to positive values of I, which has a maximum value of approximately unity. See also **rank adjacency statistic**.

Morbidity: A term used in epidemiological studies to describe sickness in human populations. The WHO Expert Committee on Health Statistics noted in its sixth report that morbidity could be measured in terms of three units:

- persons who were ill;
- the illnesses (periods or spells of illness) that those persons experienced;
- the duration of these illnesses.

Mortality: A term used in studies in *epidemiology* to describe death in human populations. Statistics on mortality are compiled from the information contained in death certificates.

Mortality odds ratio: The ratio of the observed number of deaths from a particular cause to its *expected value*, based on an assumption of equal mortality rates in the putative and comparison populations.

Mortality rate: Synonym for **death rate**.

Mosaic displays: Graphical displays of *contingency tables* in which the counts in each cell are represented by 'tiles' whose size is proportional to the cell count. See also **correspondence analysis**.

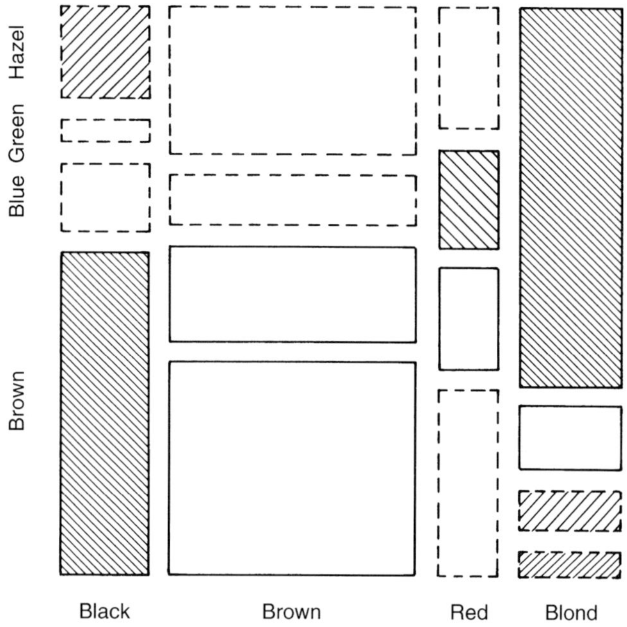

Fig 45 A mosaic display of eye colour and hair colour, in which deviations from independence are shown by shading.

Most powerful test: A test of a *null hypothesis* which has greater *power* than any other test for a given *alternative hypothesis*.

Most probable number: See **serial dilution assay**.

Mover–stayer model: A generalization of the *Markov chain model*. The basic idea is that there are two populations in the sample: stayers, who always remain in their initial state; and movers, whose transitions between states are governed by a Markov chain process.

Moving average: A method used primarily for the *smoothing* of *time series*, in which each observation is replaced by a *weighted average* of the observation and its near neighbours.

Moving average model: A *time series* having the form

$$x_t = a_t - \theta_1 a_{t-1} - \theta_2 a_{t-2} - \cdots - \theta_p a_{t-p}$$

where $a_t, a_{t-1}, \cdots, a_{t-p}$ are a *white noise sequence* and $\theta_1, \theta_2, \cdots, \theta_p$ are the parameters of the model.

MTMM: Abbreviation for **multitrait–multimethod model**.

Multicentre study: A *clinical trial* conducted simultaneously in a number of participating hospitals or clinics, with all centres following an agreed-upon study *protocol* and with independent *random allocation* within each centre. The benefits of such a study include the ability to generalize results to a wider variety of patients and treatment settings than would be possible with a study conducted in a single centre, and the ability to enrol into the study more patients than a single centre could provide.

Multicollinearity: A term used in *regression analysis* to indicate situations where the explanatory variables are related by a *linear function*, making the estimation of *regression coefficients* impossible. Including the sum of the explanatory variables in the regression analysis would, for example, lead to this problem. Approximate multicollinearity can also cause problems when estimating regression coefficients. In particular, if the *multiple correlation coefficient* for the regression of a particular explanatory variable on the others is high, then the variance of the corresponding estimated regression coefficient will also be high. See also **ridge regression**.

Multidimensional scaling: A generic term for a class of techniques that attempt to construct a low-dimensional representation of a set of observed *similarity coefficients* or *dissimilarity coefficients*, with the aim of making any structure in the data as evident as possible. See also **individual differences scaling** and **non-metric scaling**.

Multiepisode models: Models for *event history data* in which each individual may undergo more than one transition, for example, lengths of spells of unemployment or time period before moving to another region.

Multi-hit model: A model for a toxic response that results from the random occurrence of one or more fundamental biological events. A response is assumed to be induced once the target tissue has been 'hit' by a number, k, of biologically effective units of dose within a specified time period. Assuming that the number of hits during this period follows a *Poisson process*, the probability of a response is given by

$$P(\text{response}) = P(\text{at least } k \text{ hits}) = 1 - \sum_{j=0}^{k-1} \exp(-\lambda)\frac{\lambda^j}{j!}$$

where λ is the expected number of hits during this period. When $k = 1$, the multi-hit model reduces to the *one-hit model*, given by

$$P(\text{response}) = 1 - e^{-\lambda}$$

Multilevel models: Models for data that are organized hierarchically, for example, children within families, that allow for the possibility that measurements made on children from the same family are likely to be correlated.

Multimodal distribution: A *probability distribution* or *frequency distribution* with several modes. Multimodality is often taken as an indication that the observed distribution results from the mixing of the distributions of relatively distinct groups of observations. See also **finite mixture distribution**.

Multinomial distribution: A generalization of the *binomial distribution* to situations in which r outcomes can occur on each of n trials, where $r > 2$. Specifically, the distribution is given by

$$P(n_1, n_2, \cdots, n_r) = \frac{n!}{n_1!n_2!\cdots n_r!} p_1^{n_1} p_2^{n_2} \cdots p_r^{n_r}$$

where n_i is the number of trials with outcome i, and p_i is the probability of outcome i occurring on a particular trial. The *expected value* of n_i is np_i and its variance is $np_i(1 - p_i)$. The *covariance* of n_i and n_j is $-np_ip_j$.

Multiphasic screening: A process in which tests in *screening studies* may be performed in combination. For example, in cancer screening, two or more anatomic sites may be screened for cancer by tests applied to an individual during a single screening session.

Multiple comparison tests: Procedures for detailed examination of the differences between a set of means, usually after a general hypothesis that they are all equal has been rejected. No single technique is best in all situations, and a major distinction between techniques is how they control the possible inflation of the *type I error*. See also **Bonferroni correction, Duncan's multiple range test, Scheffé's test** and **Dunnett's test**.

Multiple correlation coefficient: The correlation between the observed values of the dependent variable in a *multiple regression*, and the values predicted by the estimated regression equation. Often used as an indicator of how useful the explanatory variables are in predicting the response. The square of the multiple correlation coefficient gives the proportion of variance of the response variable that is accounted for by the explanatory variables.

Multiple endpoints: A term used to describe the variety of outcome measures used in many *clinical trials*. Typically, there are multiple ways to measure treatment success, for example, length of patient survival, percentage of patients surviving for two years, or percentage of patients experiencing tumour regression. The aim in using a variety of such measures is to gain better overall knowledge of the differences between the treatments being compared. The danger with such an approach is that the performance of multiple significance tests incurs an increased risk of a *false positive result*. See also **Bonferroni correction**.

Multiple imputation: See **imputation**.

Multiple indicator multiple cause model (MIMIC): A *structural equation model* in which there are multiple indicators and multiple causes of each *latent variable*.

Multiple regression: A term usually applied to models in which a continuous response variable, y, is regressed on a number of explanatory variables, $x_1, x_2, \cdots, x_q$. Explicitly, the model fitted is

$$E(y) = \beta_0 + \beta_1 x_1 + \cdots + \beta_q x_q$$

where E denotes *expected value*. The parameters in the model, the *regression coefficients* $\beta_0, \beta_1, \cdots, \beta_q$, are generally estimated by *least squares estimation*. Each coefficient gives the change in the response variable corresponding to a unit change in the appropriate explanatory variable, conditional on the other variables remaining constant. Significance tests of whether the coefficients take the value zero can be derived on the assumption that, for a given set of values of the explanatory variables, y has a *normal distribution* with constant variance. See also **selection methods in regression** and **beta coefficient**.

Multiplication rule for probabilities: For events A and B that are independent, the probability that both occur is the product of the separate probabilities, i.e.,

$$P(A \text{ and } B) = P(A)P(B)$$

where P denotes probability.

Multiple time response data: Data arising in studies of episodic illness, such as bladder cancer and epileptic seizures. In the former, for example, individual patients may suffer multiple bladder tumours at observed times, $t_1 < t_2 < \cdots < t_k$.

Multiplicative model: A model in which the combined effect of a number of factors, when applied together, is the product of their separate effects. See also **additive model**.

Multistage model of carcinogenesis: See **Armitage–Doll model.**

Multistage sampling: Synonym for **cluster sampling**.

Multistate models: Models that arise in the context of the study of *survival times.* The experience of a patient in such a study can be represented as a process that involves two (or more) states. In the simplest situation, at the point of entry to the study, the patient is in a state that corresponds to being alive. Patients then transfer from this 'live' state to the 'dead' state at some rate measured by the *hazard function* at a given time. More complex models will involve more states. For example, a three state model might have patients alive and tumour free, patients alive and tumour present, and the 'dead' state. See also **Markov illness–death model.**

Multitrait-multimethod model (MTMM): A form of *confirmatory factor analysis* model in which different methods of measurement are used to measure each latent variable.

Multivariate analysis: A generic term for the many methods of analysis important in investigating *multivariate data.* Examples include *cluster analysis, principal components analysis* and *factor analysis.*

Multivariate analysis of variance (MANOVA): A procedure for testing the equality of the *mean vectors* of more than two populations. The technique is directly analogous to the *analysis of variance* of *univariate data*, except that the groups are compared on q response variables simultaneously. In the univariate case, *F-tests* are used to assess the hypotheses of interest. In the multivariate case, no single *test statistic* can be constructed that is optimal in all situations. The most widely used of the available test statistics is *Wilk's lambda*, which is based on three matrices, **W** (the *within groups matrix of sums of squares and products*), **T** (the *total matrix of sums of squares and cross products*) and **B** (the *between groups matrix of sums of squares and cross products*), defined as follows

$$\mathbf{T} = \sum_{i=1}^{g}\sum_{j=1}^{n_i}(\mathbf{x}_{ij} - \bar{\mathbf{x}})(\mathbf{x}_{ij} - \bar{\mathbf{x}})'$$

$$\mathbf{W} = \sum_{i=1}^{g}\sum_{j=1}^{n_i}(\mathbf{x}_{ij} - \bar{\mathbf{x}}_i)(\mathbf{x}_{ij} - \bar{\mathbf{x}}_i)'$$

$$\mathbf{B} = \sum_{i=1}^{g} n_i(\bar{\mathbf{x}}_i - \bar{\mathbf{x}})(\bar{\mathbf{x}}_i - \bar{\mathbf{x}})'$$

where $\mathbf{x}_{ij}, i = 1, \cdots, g, \quad j = 1, \cdots, n_i$ represent the jth multivariate observation in the ith group, g is the number of groups and n_i is the number of observations in the ith group. The mean vector of the ith group is represented by $\bar{\mathbf{x}}_i$, and the mean vector of all the observations by $\bar{\mathbf{x}}$. These matrices satisfy the equation

$$\mathbf{T} = \mathbf{W} + \mathbf{B}$$

Wilk's lambda is given by the ratio of the *determinants* of **W** and **T**, i.e.,

$$\Lambda = \frac{|\mathbf{W}|}{|\mathbf{T}|} = \frac{|\mathbf{W}|}{|\mathbf{W} + \mathbf{B}|}$$

The statistic, Λ, can be transformed to give an *F*-test to assess the null hypothesis of the equality of the population mean vectors. In addition to Λ, a number of other test statistics are available:

- *Roy's largest root criterion*: the largest *eigenvalue* of $\mathbf{BW}^{-1}$;
- the *Hotelling–Lawley trace*: the sum of the eigenvalues of $\mathbf{BW}^{-1}$;
- the *Pillai–Bartlett trace*: the sum of the eigenvalues of $\mathbf{BT}^{-1}$.

It has been found that the differences in *power* between the various test statistics are generally quite small, and so in most situations which is chosen will not greatly affect conclusions.

Multivariate counting process: A *stochastic process* with k components counting the occurrences, as time passes, of k different types of events, none of which can occur simultaneously.

Multivariate data: Data for which each observation consists of values for more than one *random variable*. For example, measurements on blood pressure, temperature and heart rate for a number of subjects. Such data are usually displayed in the form of a *data matrix*, i.e.,

$$\mathbf{X} = \begin{pmatrix} x_{11} & x_{12} & \cdots & x_{1q} \\ x_{21} & x_{22} & \cdots & x_{2q} \\ \vdots & \vdots & \cdots & \vdots \\ x_{n1} & x_{n2} & \cdots & x_{nq} \end{pmatrix}$$

where n is the number of subjects, q the number of variables and x_{ij} the observation on variable j for subject i.

Multivariate distribution: The simultaneous *probability distribution* of a set of *random variables*. See also **multivariate normal distribution** and **Dirichlet distribution**.

Multivariate growth data: Data arising in studies investigating the relationships in the growth of several organs of an organism and how these relationships evolve. Such data enables biologists to examine growth gradients within an organism and use these in an aid to understanding its form, function and biological niche, as well as the role of evolution in bringing it to its present form.

Multivariate normal distribution: The *probability distribution* of a set of variables, $\mathbf{x}' = [x_1, x_2, \cdots, x_q]$, given by

$$f(x_1, x_2, \cdots, x_q) = (2\pi)^{-q/2}|\Sigma|^{-\frac{1}{2}} \exp -\tfrac{1}{2}(\mathbf{x} - \boldsymbol{\mu})'\Sigma^{-1}(\mathbf{x} - \boldsymbol{\mu})$$

where $\boldsymbol{\mu}$ is the *mean vector* of the variables and Σ is their *variance–covariance matrix*. This distribution is assumed by multivariate analysis procedures such as *multivariate analysis of variance*. See also **bivariate normal distribution**.

Multivariate probit analysis: A method for assessing the effect of explanatory variables on a set of two or more correlated binary response variables. See also **probit analysis**.

Mutation distance: A distance measure for two amino acid sequences, defined as the minimal number of nucleotides that would need to be altered in order for the gene of one sequence to code for the other.

Mutation rate: The frequency with which mutations occur per gene or per generation.

Mutually exclusive events: Events that cannot occur jointly.

MYCIN: An *expert system* developed at Stanford University to assist physicians in the diagnosis and treatment of infectious diseases.

N

NANOSTAT: An interactive computer program for carrying out statistical calculations. It includes methods such as *logistic regression, principal components analysis* and *survival analysis*. Facilities are provided for data editing and for graphics output.

National Cancer Institute standards for adverse drug reactions: A five category scale for assessing adverse drug reactions ranging from none (0), mild (1), moderate (2), severe (3), life threatening (4), death (5). Both *continuous variables*, for example, white blood count, and *categorical variables*, for example, nausea, can be converted to this grading scale.

Natural history of disease: The course of a disease when left untreated or when treated with the standard therapy.

Natural history studies: The use of data, often from hospital *databases*, to study the typical course of a disease, including the symptoms and patient characteristics that influence prognosis. Such studies help in the development of new treatments and in the design of *clinical trials* to evaluate them.

Natural-pairing: See **paired samples**.

Natural response: A response of a subject or patient that is not solely due to the stimulus to which the individual has been exposed.

Nearest-neighbour clustering: Synonym for **single linkage clustering**.

Nearest-neighbour methods: Methods of *discriminant analysis* based on studying the *training set* subjects most similar to the subject to be classified. Classification might then be decided according to a simple majority verdict amongst those most similar or 'nearest' training set subjects, i.e., a subject would be assigned to the group to which the majority of the 'neighbours' belonged. Simple nearest-neighbour methods just consider the most similar neighbour. More general methods consider the k nearest neighbours, where $k > 1$.

Necessarily empty cells: Synonym for **structural zeros**.

Negative binomial distribution: For a series of *random variables* from a *Bernoulli distribution*, the probability that the kth 'success' occurs on the xth trial, with $x = k, k+1, k+2, \cdots$. Specifically, the distribution is given by

$$P(x) = \binom{x-1}{k-1} p^k (1-p)^{x-k}$$

where p is the probability of a success on a trial. The mean of the distribution is k/p and its variance is $\frac{k}{p}(\frac{1}{p} - 1)$.

Negative predictive value: The probability that a person having a negative result on a *diagnostic test* does not have the disease. See also **positive predictive value**.

Negative skewness: See **skewness**.

Negative study: A study that does not yield a statistically significant result.

Negative synergism: See **synergism**.

Neighbourhood controls: Synonym for **community controls**.

Nelder–Mead simplex algorithm: Type of **simplex algorithm**.

Neonatal mortality rate: The number of infant deaths in the first 28 days of life in a geographical area during a time period, divided by the number of live births. It is usually expressed per 1000 live births per year. For example, the rate for mothers of age 16–19 in social class I in 1949 in the UK was 7.7 per thousand live births; in 1975 the corresponding rate was 2.1.

Nested case-control study: A commonly used design in *epidemiology*, in which a cohort is followed to identify cases of some disease of interest, and the controls are selected for each case from within the cohort for comparison of exposures. The primary advantage of this design is that the exposure information needs to be gathered for only a small proportion of the cohort members, thereby considerably reducing the data collection costs.

Nested design: A design in which levels of one or more factors are subsampled within one or more other factors so that, for example, each level of a factor B occurs at only one level of another factor A. Factor B is said to be nested within factor A. An example might be where interest centres on assessing the effect of hospital and doctor on a response variable, patient satisfaction. The doctors can only practice at one hospital so they are nested within hospitals. See also **multilevel model**.

Nested model: Synonym for **hierarchical model**.

Network: A linked set of computer systems, capable of sharing computer power and/or storage facilities.

Neural networks: See **artificial neural networks**.

Newman–Keuls test: A *multiple comparison test* used to investigate in more detail the differences existing between a set of means, as indicated by a significant *F-test* in an *analysis of variance*. The test proceeds by arranging the means in increasing order and calculating the *test statistic*

$$S = \frac{\bar{x}_A - \bar{x}_B}{\sqrt{\frac{s^2}{2}\left(\frac{1}{n_A} + \frac{1}{n_B}\right)}}$$

where $\bar{x}_A$ and $\bar{x}_B$ are the two means being compared, s^2 is the *within groups mean square* from the analysis of variance, and n_A and n_B are the number of observations in the two groups. Tables of *critical values* of S are available, these depending on a parameter r that specifies the interval between the ranks of the two means being tested. For example, when comparing the largest and smallest of four means, $r = 4$, and when comparing the second smallest and smallest means, $r = 2$.

Newton–Raphson method: A numerical iterative procedure that can be used to solve non-linear equations. Often used in *maximum likelihood estimation*. If $f(x) = 0$ is the equation to be solved for x, then each iteration of the method consists of finding a closer approximation to the solution, beginning from an initial estimate $\hat{x}_0$. The $(k + 1)$th approximation is given by

$$\hat{x}_{k+1} = \hat{x}_k - f(\hat{x}_k)/f'(\hat{x}_k)$$

where $f'(\hat{x}_k)$ is the first derivative of $f(x)$ evaluated at $x = \hat{x}_k$. The iterations terminate at iteration r for which $f(\hat{x}_r)$ is close enough to zero, or the difference between $\hat{x}_k$ and $\hat{x}_{k+1}$ is negligible.

NOEL: Abbreviation for **no-observed-effect level**.

N of 1 clinical trial: A special case of a *crossover design* aimed at determining the efficacy of a treatment (or the relative merits of alternative treatments) for a specific patient. The patient is repeatedly given a treatment and placebo, or different treatments, in successive time periods. See also **interrupted time series design**.

Noise: A *stochastic process* of irregular fluctuations. See also **white noise sequence**.

Nominal significance level: The significance level of a test when its assumptions are valid.

Nominal variable: Synonym for **categorical variable**.

Nomograms: Graphic methods that permit the representation of more than two quantities on a plane surface. The example shown is of such a chart for calculating sample size or power.

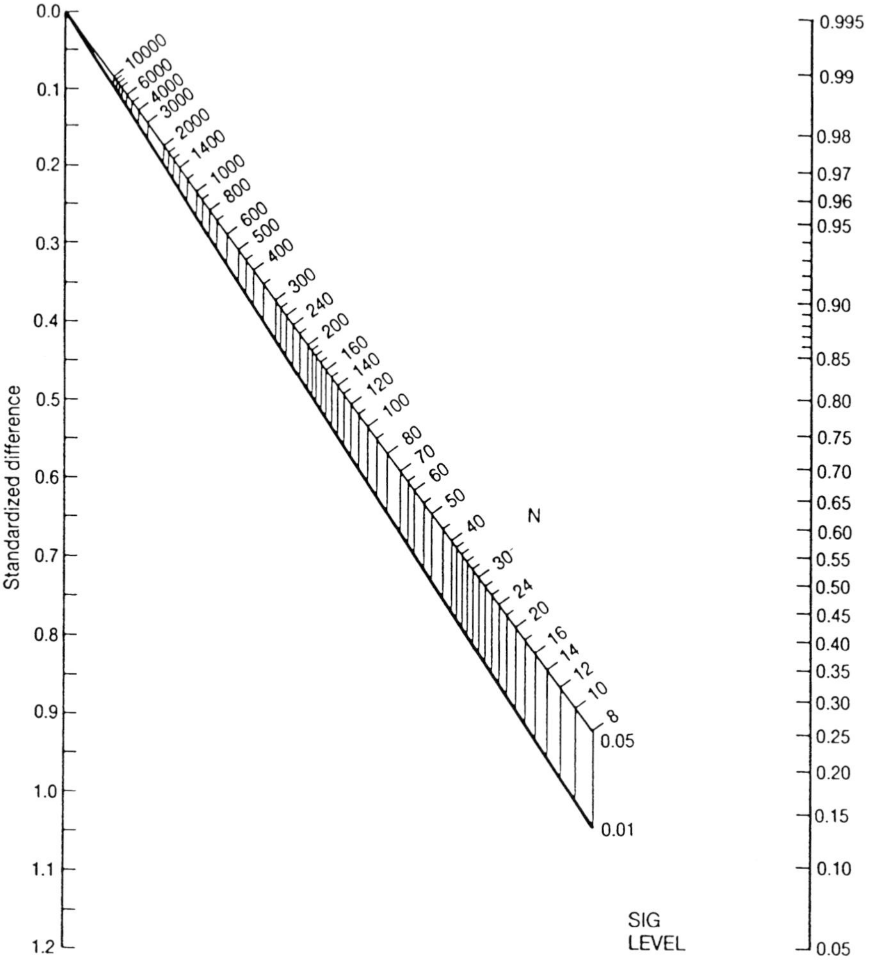

Fig 46 A nomogram for calculating sample size.

Non-central distributions: A series of *probability distributions*, each of which is an adaptation of one of the standard *sampling distributions* such as the *chi-squared distribution*, the *F-distribution* or *Student's t-distribution*. Such distributions allow the *power* of the corresponding hypothesis tests to be calculated.

Non-compliance: See **protocol violations**.

Non-current prospective study: An investigation which uses past records of both exposure to a possible risk factor and subsequent development or otherwise of some disease of interest, to avoid the costly longitudinal component of the usual type of *prospective study*. The price for this convenience is both greater chance for *bias* (including in some instances uncertainty that exposure preceeded disease), and potential knowledge of disease status when selecting for exposure.

Non-identified response: A term used to denote *censored observations* in *survival time* data, that are not independent of the endpoint of interest. Such observations can occur for a variety of reasons:

- misclassification of the response: e.g., death from cancer, the response of interest, being erroneously misclassified as death from another unrelated cause;
- response occurrence causing prior censoring: e.g., relapse to heroin use causing a subject to quit a rehabilitation study to avoid chemical detection.

Non-informative censoring: *Censored observations* that can be considered to have the same probabilities of failure at later times as those individuals remaining under observation.

Non-linear model: A model that is non-linear in the parameters, for example

$$y = \beta_1 e^{\beta_2 x_1} + \beta_3 e^{\beta_4 x_2}$$
$$y = \beta_1 e^{-\beta_2 x}$$

Some such models can be converted into *linear models* by *linearization* (the second equation above, for example, by taking logarithms throughout). Those that cannot are often referred to as *intrinsically non-linear*, although these can be approximated by linear equations in some circumstances.

Non-masked study: Synonym for **open label study**.

Non-metric scaling: A form of *multidimensional scaling* in which only the ranks of the observed *dissimilarity coefficients* or *similarity coefficients* are used in producing the required low-dimensional representation of the data. See also **monotonic regression**.

Non-orthogonal designs: *Analysis of variance* designs with two or more factors, in which the number of observations in each cell are not equal.

Non-parametric methods: See **distribution-free methods**.

Non-randomized clinical trial: A trial in which a series of consecutive patients receive a new treatment and those that respond (according to some pre-defined criterion) continue to receive it. Those patients that fail to respond receive an alternative, usually the conventional, treatment. The two groups are then compared on one or more outcome variables. One of the problems with such a procedure is that patients who respond may be healthier than those who do not respond, possibly resulting in an apparent but not real benefit of the treatment.

Non-response: A term generally used for failure to provide the relevant information being collected in a survey. Poor response can be due to a variety of causes, for example, if the topic of the survey is of an intimate nature, respondents may not care to answer particular questions. Since it is quite possible that respondents in a survey differ in some of their characteristics from those who do not respond, a large number of non-respondents may introduce *bias* into the final results. See also **item non-response**.

No-observed-effect level (NOEL): The dose level of a compound below which there is no evidence of an effect on the response of interest.

Norm: Most commonly used to refer to 'what is usual', for example, the range into which body temperatures of healthy adults fall, but also occasionally used for 'what is desirable', for example, the range of blood pressures regarded as being indicative of good health.

Normal approximation: A *normal distribution* with mean np and variance $np(1-p)$ that acts as an approximation to a *binomial distribution* as n, the number of trials, increases. The term p represents the probability of a 'success' on any trial.

Normal deviate: A value, x_p, corresponding to a proportion, p, that satisfies the following equation:

$$\int_{-\infty}^{x_p} \frac{1}{\sqrt{2\pi}} e^{-\frac{1}{2}u^2} du = p$$

Also known as the *normit*. See also **probit analysis**.

Normal distribution: A *probability distribution* of a *random variable*, x, that is assumed by many statistical methods. Specifically given by

$$f(x) = \frac{1}{\sigma\sqrt{2\pi}} \exp\left[-\frac{1}{2}\frac{(x-\mu)^2}{\sigma^2}\right]$$

where μ and σ^2 are, respectively, the mean and variance of x. This distribution is *bell-shaped*, as shown in the example.

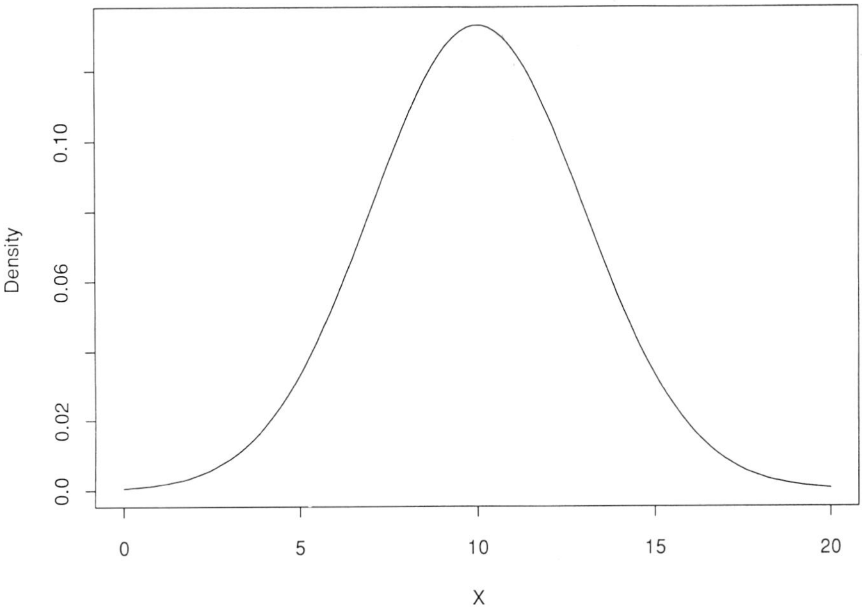

Fig 47 A normal distribution with mean = 10 and variance = 9.

Normality: A term used to indicate that some variable of interest has a *normal distribution.*

Normal probability plot: See **quantile–quantile plot**.

Normal range: Synonym for **reference interval**.

Normit: See **normal equivalent deviate**.

NORMIX: A computer program for the *maximum likelihood estimation* of the parameters in a *finite mixture distribution* in which the components are *multivariate normal distributions* with different *mean vectors* and possibly different *variance-covariance matrices.*

Nuisance parameter: A parameter that is needed to specify a *probability distribution*, but is not of central importance compared with others. The presence of such parameters can make testing hypotheses about those of more interest difficult, and it is often necessary to find a *test statistic* that does not depend on them. See also **likelihood**.

Null distribution: The *probability distribution* of a *test statistic* when the *null hypothesis* is true.

Null hypothesis (H_0): The 'no difference' or 'no association' hypothesis to be tested (usually by means of a significance test) against an *alternative hypothesis* that postulates non-zero difference or association.

Null matrix: A *matrix* in which all elements are zero.

Null vector: A *vector*, the elements of which are all zero.

Numerical taxonomy: In essence, a synonym for **cluster analysis**.

Nyquist frequency: A term applied to *time series* data where the observations are recorded at equal intervals, to denote the frequency of a cyclical term whose period is twice the time interval between successive observations.

O

Oblique factors: A term used in *factor analysis* for *common factors* that are allowed to be correlated.

O'Brien's two-sample tests: Extensions of the conventional tests for assessing differences between treatment groups, that take account of the possible heterogeneous nature of the response to treatment, and which may be useful in the identification of subgroups of patients for whom the experimental therapy might have most (or least) benefit.

Observational study: A general term for investigations in which the researcher has little or no control over events, and the relationships between *risk factors* and outcome measures are studied without the intervention of the investigator. Surveys and most studies in *epidemiology* fall into this class. See also **experimental study, prospective study**, and **retrospective study**.

Occam's razor: An early statement of the *parsimony principle*, namely 'entia non sunt multiplicanda praeter necessitatem'.

Occupational death rates: Mortality rates calculated within occupational categories. See also **age-specific death rate** and **cause-specific death rate**.

Odds: The ratio of the probabilities of the two possible states of a *binary variable*. See also **odds ratio** and **logistic regression**.

Odds ratio: The ratio of the *odds* for a *binary variable* in two groups of subjects, for example, males and females. If the two possible states of the variable are labelled 'success' and 'failure', then the odds ratio is a measure of the odds of a success in one group relative to that in the other. When the odds of a success in each group are identical then the odds ratio is equal to unity. Usually estimated as

$$\hat{\psi} = \frac{ad}{bc}$$

where a, b, c and d are the appropriate frequencies in the *two-by-two contingency table* formed from the data. See also **Haldane's estimator, Jewell's estimator** and **logistic regression**.

Offset: A term used in *generalized linear models* to indicate a known *regression coefficient* that is to be included in a model, i.e., one that does not have to be estimated. For example, suppose the number of deaths for district i and age class j is assumed to follow a *Poisson distribution* with mean $N_{ij}\theta_{ij}$, where N_{ij} is the total person years for district i and age class j. Further, it is postulated that the parameter θ_{ij} is the product of district (θ_i) and age (θ_j) effects. The model for the mean (μ) is thus

$$\ln(\mu) = \ln(N_{ij}) + \ln\theta_i + \ln\theta_j$$

The first term on the right hand side is the offset.

Ogive: A term often applied to the graphs of *cumulative frequency distributions*. Essentially synonymous with *sigmoid*, which is to be preferred.

OLS: Abbreviation for **ordinary least squares**.

Omitted covariates: A term usually found in connection with *generalized linear models*, where the model has been incompletely specified by not including important covariates. In observational studies, for example, the omission may be due either to an incorrect conceptual understanding of the phenomena under study or to an inability to collect data on all the relevant factors related to the outcome under study. Mis-specifying generalized linear models in this way can result in seriously biased estimates of the effects of the covariates actually included in the model.

One-hit model: See **multi-hit model**.

One:*m* (1:*m*) matching: A form of *matching* often used when control subjects are more readily obtained than cases. A number, m ($m > 1$), of controls are attached to each case, these being known as the *matched set*. The theoretical efficiency of such matching in estimating, for example, *relative risk*, is $m/(m+1)$, so one control per case is 50% efficient, while four per case is 80% efficient. Increasing the number of controls beyond 5–10 brings rapidly diminishing returns.

One-sided test: A significance test for which the *alternative hypothesis* is directional; for example, that one population mean is greater than another. The choice between a one-sided and *two-sided test* must be made before any *test statistic* is calculated.

One-step method: A procedure for obtaining a pooled estimate of an *odds ratio* from a set of *two-by-two contingency tables*. Not recommended for general use, since it can lead to extremely biased results, particularly when applied to unbalanced data. The *Mantel–Haenszel estimator* is usually far more satisfactory.

One-tailed test: Synonym for **one-sided test**.

One way design: See **analysis of variance**.

Open label study: An investigation in which patient, investigator and peripheral staff are all aware of what treatment the patient is receiving.

Open sequential design: See **sequential analysis**.

Operational research: Research concerned with applying scientific methods to the problems facing executive and administrative authorities.

Opinion survey: A procedure that aims to ascertain opinions possessed by members of some population with regard to particular topics. See also **sample survey**.

Optimization methods: Procedures for finding the maxima or minima of functions of, generally, several variables. Most often encountered in statistics in the context of *maximum likelihood estimation*, where such methods are frequently needed to find the values of the parameters that maximize the *likelihood*. See also **simplex method** and **Newton–Raphson method**.

Option-3 scheme: A scheme of measurement used in situations investigating possible changes over time in *longitudinal data*. The scheme is designed to prevent measurement *outliers* causing an unexpected increase in falsely claiming that a change in the data has occurred. Two measures are taken initially and, if they are closer than a specified threshold, the average of the two is considered to be an estimate of the true mean; otherwise a third measurement is made, and the mean of the closest 'pair' is considered to be the estimate.

Ordered alternative hypothesis: A hypothesis that specifies an order for a set of parameters of interest as an alternative to their equality, rather than simply that they are not all equal. For example, in an evaluation of the treatment effect of a drug at several different doses, it might be thought reasonable to postulate that the response variable shows either a *monotonic increasing* or *monotonic decreasing* effect with dose. In such a case the *null hypothesis* of the equality of, say, a set of m means would be tested against

$$\mathrm{H}_1 : \mu_1 \leq \mu_2 \cdots \leq \mu_m,$$

using some suitable test procedure such as *Jonckheere's k-sample test*.

Order statistics: Particular values in a ranked set of observations. The rth largest value in a sample, for example, is called the rth order statistic.

Ordinal variable: A measurement that allows a sample of individuals to be ranked with respect to some characteristic, but where differences at different points of the scale are not necessarily equivalent. For example, anxiety might be rated on a scale 'none', 'mild', 'moderate' and 'severe', with the values 0,1,2,3, being used to label the categories. A patient with anxiety score of 1 could be ranked as less anxious than one given a score of 3, but patients with scores 0 and 2 do not necessarily have the same difference in anxiety as patients with scores 1 and 3. See also **categorical variable** and **continuous variable**.

Ordinary least squares (OLS): See **least squares estimation**.

Ordination: The process of reducing the dimensionality (i.e., the number of variables) of *multivariate data* by deriving a small number of new variables that contain much of the information in the original data. The reduced data set is often more useful for investigating possible structure in the observations. See also **principal components analysis** and **multidimensional scaling**.

Orthogonal: A term that occurs in several areas of statistics with different meanings in each case. Most commonly encountered in relation to two variables or two *linear functions* of a set of variables to indicate statistical independence. Literally means 'at right angles'.

Orthogonal contrasts: Sets of *linear functions* of either parameters or statistics in which the defining coefficients satisfy a particular relationship. Specifically, if c_1 and c_2 are two *contrasts* of a set of m parameters such that

$$c_1 = a_{11}\beta_1 + a_{12}\beta_2 + \cdots + a_{1m}\beta_m$$
$$c_2 = a_{21}\beta_1 + a_{22}\beta_2 + \cdots + a_{2m}\beta_m$$

they are orthogonal if $\sum_{i=1}^{m} a_{1i}a_{2i} = 0$. If, in addition, $\sum_{i=1}^{m} a_{1i}^2 = 1$ and $\sum_{i=1}^{m} a_{2i}^2 = 1$, then the contrasts are said to be *orthonormal*.

Orthogonal matrix: A *square matrix* that is such that multiplying the matrix by its transpose results in an *identity matrix*.

Orthonormal contrasts: See **orthogonal contrasts**.

Outcome variable: Synonym for **response variable**.

Outlier: An observation that appears to deviate markedly from the other members of the sample in which it occurs. In the set of systolic blood pressures, $\{125, 128, 130, 131, 198\}$, for example, 198 might be considered an outlier. Such extreme observations may be reflecting some abnormality in the measured characteristic of a patient, or they may result from an error in the measurement or recording. See also **log-likelihood distance, outside observation**, **five-number summary** and **Wilk's multivariate outlier test**.

Outside observation: An observation falling outside the limits

$$F_L - 1.5(F_U - F_L), F_U + 1.5(F_U - F_L)$$

where F_U and F_L are the upper and lower quartiles of a sample. Such observations are usually regarded as being extreme enough to be potential *outliers*. See also **box-and-whisker plot**.

Overdispersion: A phenomenon encountered when modelling data that occurs in the form of proportions, where it is often observed that there is more variation than, for example, an assumed *binomial distribution* can accomodate. There may be a variety of relatively simple causes of the increased variation, ranging from the presence of one or more *outliers*, to *misspecification* of the model being applied to the data. If none of these explanations can explain the phenomenon, then it is likely that it is due to variation between the response probabilities or correlation between the binary responses, in which case special modelling procedures may be needed. See also **clustered binary data** and **generalized linear model**.

Overfitted models: Models that contain more unknown parameters than can be justified by the data.

Overidentified model: See **identification**.

Overmatching: A term applied to studies involving *matching* when the matching variable is strongly related to exposure but not to disease risk. Such a situation leads to a loss of efficiency.

Overparameterized model: A model with more parameters than observations for estimation. For example, the following simple model for a *one way design* in *analysis of variance*:

$$y_{ij} = \mu + \alpha_i + e_{ij} \qquad (i = 1, 2, \cdots, g; j = 1, 2, \cdots, n_i)$$

where g is the number of groups, n_i the number of observations in group i, y_{ij} represents the jth observation in the ith group, μ is the grand mean effect and α_i the effect of group i, has $g + 1$ parameters but only g group means to be fitted. It is overparameterized unless some constraints are placed on the parameters, for example, that $\sum_{i=1}^{g} \alpha_i = 0$. See also **identification**.

Overviews: Synonym for **meta-analysis**.

P

Paired availability design: A design which can reduce *selection bias* in situations where it is not possible to use *random allocation* of subjects to treatments. The design has three fundamental characteristics:

- the intervention is the availability of treatment, not its receipt;
- the population from which subjects arise is well defined with little in- or out-migration;
- the study involves many pairs of control and experimental groups.

In the experimental groups, the new treatment is made available to all subjects, though some may not receive it. In the control groups, the experimental treatment is generally not available to subjects, though some may receive it in special circumstances.

Paired Bernoulli data: Data arising when an investigator records whether a particular characteristic is present or absent at two sites on the same individual.

Paired samples: Two samples of observations with the characteristic feature that each observation in one sample has one and only one matching observation in the other sample. There are several ways in which such samples can arise in medical investigations. The first, *self-pairing*, occurs when each subject serves as his or her own control, as in, for example, therapeutic trials in which each subject receives both treatments, one on each of two separate occasions. Next, *natural-pairing* can arise, particularly, for example, in laboratory experiments involving litter-mate controls. Lastly, *artificial pairing* may be used by an investigator to match the two subjects in a pair on important characteristics likely to be related to the response variable.

Paired samples t-test: Synonym for **matched pairs t-test**.

Pandemic: An epidemic occurring over a very wide area and usually affecting a large proportion of the population.

Panel study: A study in which a group of people, the 'panel', are interviewed or surveyed with respect to some topic of interest on more than one occasion.

Essentially equivalent to a *longitudinal study*, although there may be many response variables observed at each time point.

Parallel distributed processing (PDP): Information processing involving a large number of units working contemporaneously in parallel with units, like the neurons of the brain, exciting or inhibiting one another. See also **artificial neural networks**.

Parallel-dose design: See **dose-ranging trial**.

Parallel groups design: A simple experimental setup in which two different groups of patients, for example, treated and untreated, are studied concurrently.

Parallelism in ANCOVA: One of the assumptions made in the *analysis of covariance*, namely, that the slope of the regression line relating the response variable to the covariate is the same in all treatment groups.

Parallel-line bioassay: A procedure for estimating *equipotent doses*. The model used can be formulated by the following equations:

$$y_s = \alpha + \beta x_s$$
$$y_t = \alpha + \beta(x_t + \mu)$$

where y_s, y_t are the responses to doses x_s, x_t (usually transformed in terms of logarithms to base 10) involving a known standard preparation against a test preparation, respectively. The objective is to estimate the relative potency, ρ, of the test preparation, where $\log \rho = \mu$, i.e., the horizontal shift between the parallel lines. Note that if the test preparation is as potent as the standard preparation, then $\rho = 1$ or, equivalently, $\mu = 0$.

Parameter: A numerical characteristic of a population or a model. The probability of a 'success' in a *binomial distribution*, for example.

Parametric hypothesis: A hypothesis concerning the parameter(s) of a distribution. For example, the hypothesis that the mean of a population equals the mean of a second population, when the populations are each assumed to have a *normal distribution*.

Parametric methods: Procedures for testing hypotheses about parameters in a population described by a specified distributional form, often a *normal distribution*. *Student's t-test* is an example of such a method. See also **distribution-free methods**.

Parallel coordinate plots: A simple but powerful technique for obtaining a graphical display of *multivariate data*. In this plot, the variable axes are arranged horizontally, each parallel to the one above it. A line is then plotted for

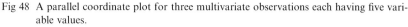

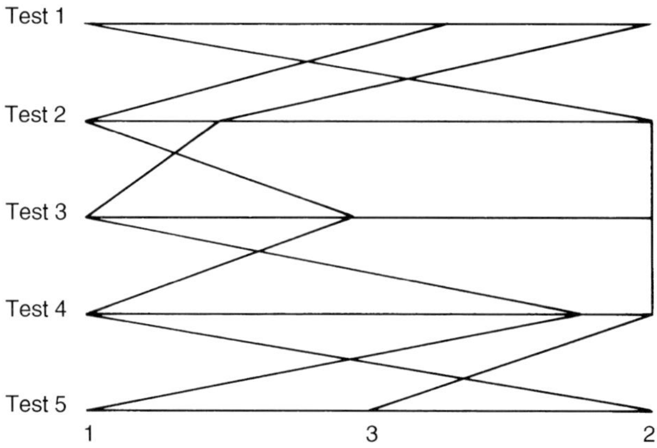

Fig 48 A parallel coordinate plot for three multivariate observations each having five variable values.

each observation by joining the appropriate variable values on these axes. The example given shows such a plot for three observations, each with five variable values. See also **Andrew's plots** and **Chernoff's faces**.

Parsimony principle: The general principle that amongst competing models, all of which provide an adequate fit for a set of data, the one with the fewest parameters is to be preferred. See also **Occam's razor**.

Partial autocorrelation: A measure of the correlation between the observations a particular number of time units apart in a *time series*, after controlling for the effects of observations at intermediate time points.

Partial correlation: The correlation between a pair of variables after adjusting for the effect of a third. Can be calculated from the sample *correlation coefficients* of each of the three pairs of variables involved as

$$r_{12|3} = \frac{r_{12} - r_{13}r_{23}}{\sqrt{(1 - r_{13}^2)(1 - r_{23}^2)}}$$

As an example, consider the correlation between dizygotic (Dz) twinning rate and latitude, which for 19 European countries has been calculated as 0.68. The correlation between milk consumption and latitude is 0.92, and between milk consumption and Dz twinning rate it is 0.61. The partial correlation between latitude and Dz twinning rate is therefore 0.18. This small value suggests that one possible explanation for the relatively high observed correlation between Dz twinning rate and latitude might be milk consumption.

Partial multiple correlation coefficient: An index for examining the linear relationship between a response variable, y, and a group of explanatory variables,

$x_1, x_2, \cdots, x_k$, whilst controlling for a further group of variables, $x_{k+1}, x_{k+2}, \cdots, x_q$. Specifically given by the *multiple correlation coefficient* of the variable $y - \hat{y}$ and the variables $x_1 - \hat{x}_1, x_2 - \hat{x}_2, \cdots, x_k - \hat{x}_k$, where the 'hats' indicate the predicted value of a variable from its linear regression on $x_{k+1}, x_{k+2}, \cdots, x_q$.

Partial questionnaire design: A procedure used in studies in *epidemiology*, as an alternative to a lengthy questionnaire which can result in lower rates of participation by potential study subjects. Information about the exposure of interest is obtained from all subjects, but information about secondary variables is determined for only a fraction of study subjects.

Partial-regression leverage plot: Synonym for **added variable plot**.

Partner studies: Studies involving pairs of individuals living together. Such studies are often particularly useful for estimating the *transmission probabilities* of infectious diseases.

Passenger variable: A term occasionally used for a variable, A, that is associated with another variable B only because of their separate relationships to a third variable C.

Path analysis: A tool for evaluating the interrelationships among variables by analysing their correlational structure. The relationships between the variables are often illustrated graphically by means of a *path diagram*, in which single headed arrows indicate the direct influence of one variable on another, and curved double headed arrows indicate correlated variables. Originally introduced for simple regression models for observed variables, the method has now become the basis for more sophisticated procedures such as *confirmatory factor analysis* and *structural equation modelling*, involving both *manifest variables* and *latent variables*.

Path coefficient: Synonym for **standardized regression coefficient**.

Path diagram: See **path analysis**. (See Fig. 49 overleaf.)

Patient time: A term sometimes used for the period of time a patient spends in a study.

Pattern recognition: A term used primarily in electrical engineering for *classification techniques*. *Unsupervised pattern recognition* is synonymous with *cluster analysis*. *Supervised pattern recognition* is synonymous with *discriminant analysis*.

PDP: Abbreviation for **parallel distributed processing**.

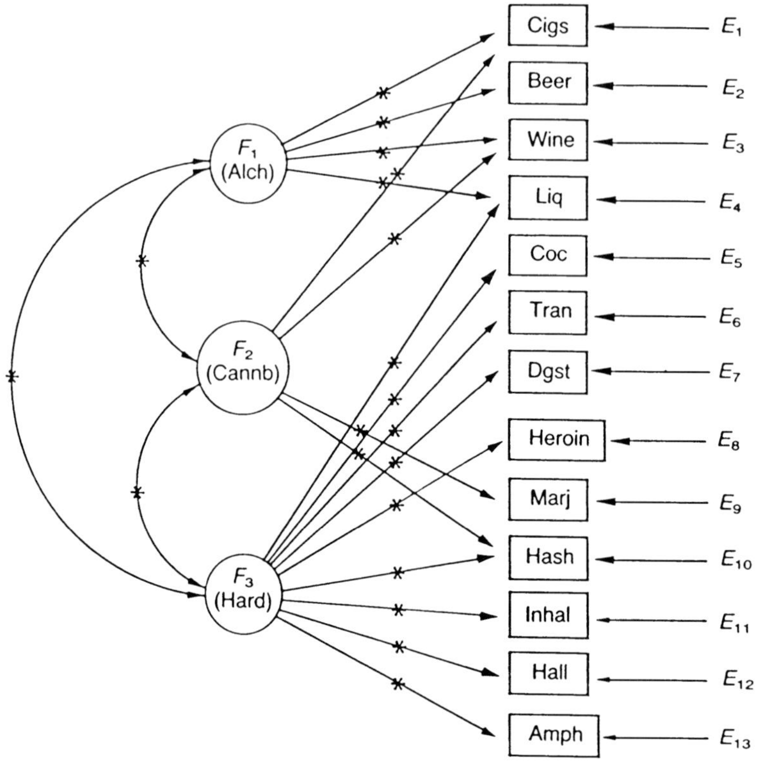

Fig 49 A path diagram for a confirmatory factor analysis model.

Peak value: The maximum value of (usually) a *dose–response curve*. Often used as an additional (or alternative) response measure to the *area under the curve*.

Pearl rate: A method used to summarize pregnancy rates in studies of the effectiveness of contraceptives. Calculated as (number of events/number of months of exposure)×1200.

Pearson residual: A model diagnostic used particularly in the analysis of *contingency tables* and *logistic regression*, and given by

$$r_i = \frac{O_i - E_i}{\sqrt{E_i}}$$

where O_i represents the observed value and E_i the corresponding predicted value under some model. Such residuals, if the assumed model is true, have approximately a *standard normal distribution*, and so values outside the range -2.0 to 2.0 suggest aspects of the current model that are inadequate.

Pearson's chi-squared statistic: See **chi-squared statistic**.

Pearson's product moment correlation coefficient: See **correlation coefficient**.

Pedigree: A term used in genetics for any grouping of related individuals, for example, pairs such as twins and spouses, and larger groups such as nuclear or extended families. The term does not exclude genetically unrelated persons.

Penetrance: The proportion of individuals of a specified *genotype* that show the expected *phenotype* under a defined set of environmental conditions.

Penetrance probability: The probability of disease for an individual who has a given *genotype* at the locus under study.

Percentile: The set of divisions that produce exactly 100 equal parts in a series of continuous values, such as blood pressure, weight and height. Thus, a person with blood pressure above the 80th percentile has a greater blood pressure value than over 80% of the other recorded values.

Percentile–percentile plot: Synonym for **quantile–quantile plot**.

Per-comparison error rate: The significance level at which each test or comparison is carried out in an experiment. See also **per-experiment error rate**.

Per-experiment error rate: The probability of incorrectly rejecting at least one null hypothesis in an experiment involving one or more tests or comparisons, when the corresponding *null hypothesis* is true in each case. See also **per-comparison error rate**.

Perinatal mortality rate: The number of stillbirths plus deaths in the first week of life, divided by the total number of live plus stillbirths. Usually expressed per 1000 total births per year. The following table gives the rates for England, Wales, Scotland and Northern Ireland for both 1971 and 1992.

	1971	**1992**
England	22.1	7.6
Wales	24.4	7.0
Scotland	24.5	9.0
Northern Ireland	27.2	8.0

Period: See **cycle**.

Periodic survey: Synonym for **panel study**.

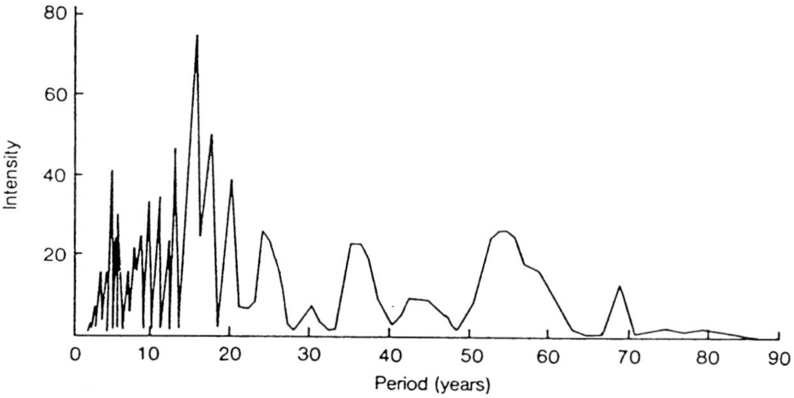

Fig 50 An example of a periodogram.

Periodogram: A graphical display used in *harmonic analysis* of *time series* data. If the value of the series at time t is u_t, the procedure involves calculating

$$A = \frac{2}{n}\sum_{t=1}^{n} u_t \cos \lambda t \quad , \quad B = \frac{2}{n}\sum_{t=1}^{n} u_t \sin \lambda t$$

and then plotting $A^2 + B^2$ (known as the intensity), against the period given by $2\pi/\lambda$. Peaks in the plot indicate periodicities in the original series. See also **spectral analysis**.

Period prevalence: See **prevalence**.

Permutation test: Synonym for **randomization test**.

Personal probabilities: A radically different approach to the allocation of probabilities than the commonly used long-term frequency method (see the entry under *Probability*). Here probability reflects subjective ignorance and knowledge which can be quantified in terms of betting behaviour. One definition offered by Savage is

> *My probability for an event* A *under circumstances* H *is the amount of money I am indifferent to betting on* A *in an elementary gambling situation.*

Person-time: A term used in studies in *epidemiology* for the total observation time added over subjects.

Person-time incidence rate: A measure of the *incidence* of an event in some population given by

$$\frac{\text{number of events occurring during the interval}}{\text{number of person-time units at risk observed during the interval}}$$

Perspective plot: See **contour plot**.

Pertubation methods: Methods for investigating the stability of statistical models when the observations suffer small random changes.

PEST: Software for the planning and application of *sequential analysis*.

Petersen estimator: See **capture–recapture sampling**.

Phase I study: Initial *clinical trials* on a new compound, usually conducted amongst healthy volunteers with a view to assessing safety.

Phase II study: Once a drug has been established as safe in a *Phase I study*, the next stage is to conduct a *clinical trial* in patients to determine the optimum dose and to assess the efficacy of the compound.

Phase III study: Large multi-centre comparative *clinical trials* to demonstrate the safety and efficacy of the new treatment with respect to the standard treatments available. These are the studies that are needed to support product licence applications.

Phase IV study: Studies conducted after a drug is marketed to provided additional details about its safety, efficacy and usage profile.

Phenotype: See **genotype**.

Phi-coefficient: A measure of association of the two variables forming a *two-by-two contingency table*, given simply by

$$\phi = \sqrt{\frac{X^2}{N}}$$

where X^2 is the usual *chi-squared statistic* for the independence of the two variables and N is the sample size. The coefficient has a maximum value of unity, and the closer its value to unity, the stronger the association between the two variables. See also **Cramer's V** and **contingency coefficient**.

Pickles charts: Day-by-day plots of new cases of infectious diseases according to their dates of onset.

Pie chart: A widely used graphical technique for presenting the distributions associated with the observed values of a *categorical variable*. The chart consists of a circle subdivided into sectors whose sizes are proportional to the quantities (usually percentages) they represent. An example is given. Such displays are popular in the media but have little relevance for ser-

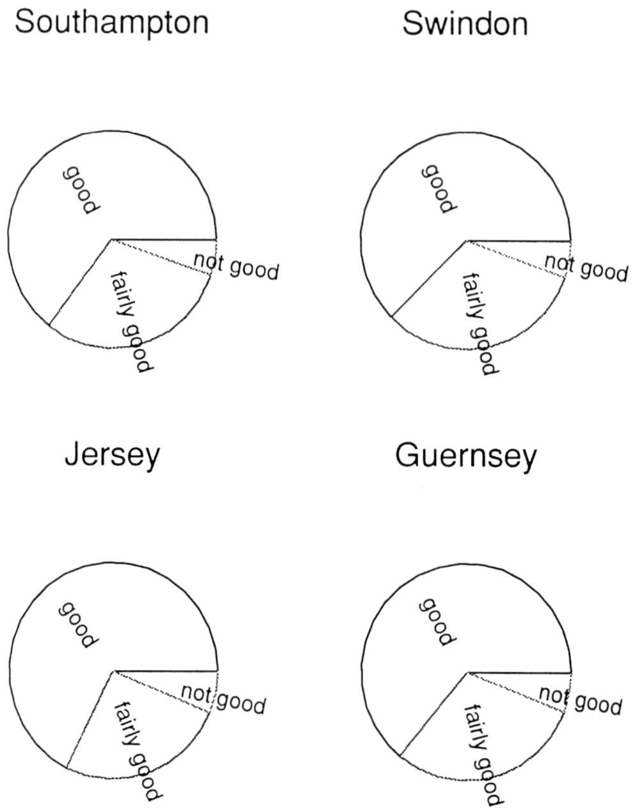

Fig 51 Pie charts for subjective assessments of health in four regions.

ious scientific work, when other graphics are generally far more useful. See also **bar chart** and **dot plot**.

Pillai–Bartlett trace: See **multivariate analysis of variance**.

Pilot study: A small scale investigation designed either to test the feasibility of methods and procedures for later use on a large scale, or to search for possible effects and associations that may be worth following up in a subsequent larger study.

Pilot survey: A small scale investigation carried out before the main survey, primarily to gain information and to identify problems relevant to the survey proper.

Pivotal variable: A function of one or more statistics and one or more parameters that has the same *probability distribution* for all values of the parameters. For example, the statistic, z, given by

$$z = \frac{\bar{x} - \mu}{\sigma/\sqrt{n}}$$

has a *standard normal distribution* whatever the values of μ and σ.

Pixel: A contraction of 'picture-element'. The smallest element of a display.

Placebo: A treatment designed to appear exactly like a comparison treatment, but which is devoid of the active component.

Placebo effect: A well-known phenomenon in medicine in which patients given only inert substances often show subsequent clinical improvement when compared with patients not so 'treated'.

Placebo reactor: A term sometimes used for those patients in a *clinical trial* who report side effects normally associated with the active treatment while receiving a placebo.

Planned comparisons: Comparisons between a set of means suggested before data are collected. Usually more powerful than a general test for mean differences.

Platykurtic curve: See **kurtosis**.

Play-the-winner rule: A procedure sometimes considered in *clinical trials* in which the response to treatment is either positive (a success) or negative (a failure). One of the two treatments is selected at random and used on the first patient; thereafter the same treatment is used on the next patient whenever the response of the previously treated patient is positive, and the other treatment whever the response is negative.

Point-biserial correlation: A special case of *Pearson's product moment correlation coefficient* used when one variable is continuous (y) and the other is a *binary variable* (x) representing a natural dichotomy. Given by

$$r_{pb} = \frac{\bar{y}_1 - \bar{y}_0}{s_y}\sqrt{pq}$$

where $\bar{y}_1$ is the sample mean of the y variable for those individuals with $x = 1$, $\bar{y}_0$ is the sample mean of the y variable for those individuals with $x = 0$, s_y is the standard deviation of the y values, p is the proportion of individuals with $x = 1$, and $q = 1 - p$ is the proportion of individuals with $x = 0$. See also **biserial correlation**.

Point estimate: See **estimate**.

Point estimation: See **estimation**.

Point prevalence: See **prevalence**.

Point process: A statistical process concerned with the occurrence of events at points of time or space determined by some chance mechanism.

Point scoring: A simple *distribution-free method* that can be used for the prediction of a response that is a *binary variable* from the observations on a number of explanatory variables which are also binary. The simplest version of the procedure, often called the *Burgess method*, operates by first taking the explanatory variables one at a time and determining which level of each variable is associated with the higher proportion of the 'success' category of the binary response. The prediction score for any individual is then just the number of explanatory variables at the high level (usually only variables that are 'significant' are included in the score). The score therefore varies from 0, when all explanatory variables are at the low level, to its maximum value when all the significant variables are at the high level. The aim of the method is to divide the population into risk groups.

Poisson distribution: The *probability distribution* of the number of occurrences of some random event, x, in an interval of time or space, and given by

$$P(x) = \frac{e^{-\lambda}\lambda^x}{x!}, x = 0, 1, \cdots$$

The mean and variance of a variable with such a distribution are both equal to λ.

Poisson homogeneity test: See **index of dispersion**.

Poisson process: A *point process* with independent increments at constant intensity, say λ. The count after time t has therefore a *Poisson distribution* with mean λt.

Polishing: An iterative process aimed at producing a set of residuals from a *linear regression* analysis that show no relationship to the explanatory variable.

Politz–Simmons technique: A method for dealing with the 'not-at-home' problem in household interview surveys. The results are weighted in accordance with the proportion of days the respondent is ordinarily at home at the time he or she was interviewed. More weight is given to respondents who are seldom at home, who represent a group with a high non-response rate.

Polyá distribution: See **beta-binomial distribution**.

Polychotomous variables: Strictly, variables that can take more than two possible values, but since this would include all but *binary variables*, the term is conventionally used for *categorical variables* with more than two categories.

Polynomial regression: A *linear model* in which powers and possibly cross-products of explanatory variables are included. For example

$$y = \beta_0 + \beta_1 x + \beta_2 x^2$$

Polynomial trend: A *trend* of the general form

$$y = \beta_0 + \beta_1 t + \beta_2 t^2 + \cdots + \beta_m t^m$$

often fitted to a *time series.*

Population: In statistics this term is used for any finite or infinite collection of 'units', which are often people, but may be, for example, institutions, events, etc. See also **sample**.

Population averaged models: Models used in the analysis of *clustered binary data* in which the *expected value* of a response variable is modelled as a function of covariates, and some working covariance structure is used to account for *intraclass correlation.* An example is the *generalized estimating equation* approach as used in the analysis of *longitudinal studies* with such variables. See also **cluster-specific models** and **mixed effects logistic regression**.

Population projection matrix: See **Leslie matrix model**.

Population pyramid: A diagram designed to show the comparison of a human population by sex and age at a given time, consisting of a pair of histograms, one for each sex, laid on their sides with a common base. The diagram is intended to provide a quick overall comparison of the age and sex structure of the population. A population whose pyramid has a broad base and narrow apex has high fertility. Changing shape over time reflects the changing composition of the population associated with changes in fertility and mortality at each age. The example given overleaf shows such diagrams for two countries with very different age/sex compositions.

Positive predictive value: The probability that a person having a positive result on a *diagnostic test* actually has a particular disease. See also **negative predictive value**.

Positive skewness: See **skewness**.

Positive synergism: See **synergism**.

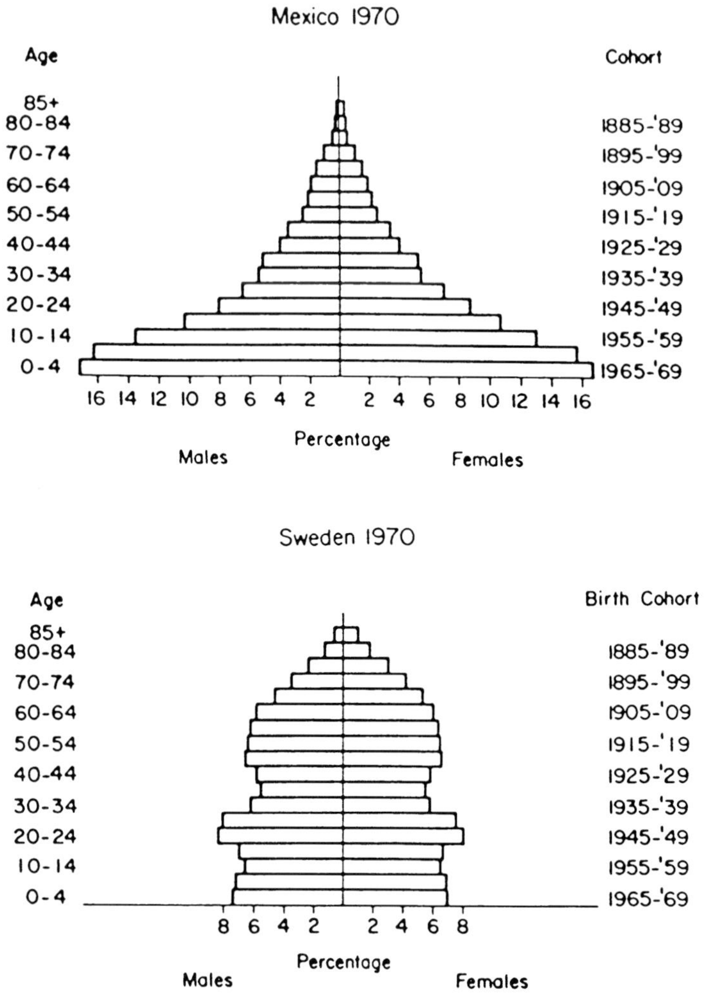

Fig 52 Population pyramids for two countries.

Posterior distributions: *Probability distributions* that summarize information about a *random variable* or parameter after, or *a posterior* to, having obtained new information from empirical data. Used almost entirely within the context of *Bayesian inference*. See also **prior distributions**.

Posterior probability: See **Bayes' theorem**.

Post-hoc comparisons: Analyses not explicitly planned at the start of a study but suggested by an examination of the data. See also **multiple comparison tests, subgroup analysis, data dredging** and **planned comparisons**.

Post-neonatal mortality rate: The number of infant deaths between the 29th day and the end of the first year of life, divided by the number of live births in the same time period. Usually expressed per 1000 live births per year.

Poststratification: The classification of a simple *random sample* of individuals into *strata* after selection. In contrast to a conventional *stratified random sampling*, the stratum sizes are here *random variables*.

Potency index: An index used to provide a ranking of animal carcinogens, given by

$$C_q = K - \log_{10} d_q$$

where the constant K is usually set to 7, so that the index will generally be in the range 1–10. The term d_q is the dose (in μmol/kg body weight per day) obtained from the *dose–response curve* corresponding to *quantile* q, usually chosen in the range 0.10–0.50.

Power: The probability of rejecting the *null hypothesis* when it is false. Power gives a method of discriminating between competing tests of the same hypothesis, the test with the higher power being preferred. It is also the basis of procedures for estimating the sample size needed to detect an effect of a particular magnitude.

Power transformation: A transformation of the form $y = x^m$.

Pragmatic trial: A *clinical trial* in which the primary objective is to be able to make explicit recommendations concerning patients in the future.

Precision: A term applied to the likely spread of estimates of a parameter in a statistical model. Measured by the *standard error* of the estimator; this can be decreased, and hence precision increased, by using a larger sample size.

Predictor variables: Synonym for **explanatory variables**.

Prescription sequence analysis: A procedure which use pharmacy-based prescription drug histories to detect a subset of drug effects.

PRESS statistic: A measure of the generalizability of a model in a *regression analysis*, based on the calculation of residuals of the form

$$\hat{e}_{(-i)} = y_i - \hat{y}_{(-i)}$$

where y_i is the observed value of the response variable for observation i and $\hat{y}_{(-i)}$ is the predicted value of the response variable for this observation, found from the fitted regression equation calculated from the data after omitting the observation. From these residuals a *multiple correlation* type statistic is obtained as

$$R^2_{\text{PRESS}} = 1 - \sum_{i=1}^{n} \hat{e}^2_{(-i)} \Big/ \sum_{i=1}^{n} (y_i - \bar{y})^2$$

This can be used to assess competing models.

Prevalence: A measure of the number of people in a population who have a particular disease at a given point in time. Can be measured in two ways, as *point prevalence* and *period prevalence*, these being defined as follows:

$$\text{point prevalence} = \frac{\text{number of cases at a particular moment}}{\text{number in population at that moment}}$$

$$\text{period prevalence} = \frac{\text{number of cases during a specified time period}}{\text{number in population at midpoint of period}}$$

Essentially measures the existence of a disease. See also **incidence**.

Prevented fraction: A measure that can be used to attribute protection against disease directly to an intervention. The measure is given by the proportion of disease that would have occurred had the intervention not been present in the population, i.e.,

$$\text{PF} = \frac{\text{PAI} - \text{PI}}{\text{PAI}}$$

where PAI is the risk of disease in the absence of the intervention in the population and PI is overall risk in the presence of the intervention. See also **attributable risk**.

Prevention trials: *Clinical trials* designed to test treatments preventing the onset of disease in healthy subjects. An early example of such a trial was that involving various whooping-cough vaccines in the 1940s.

Principal components analysis: A procedure for analysing *multivariate data*, which transforms the original variables into new ones that are uncorrelated and account for decreasing proportions of the variance in the data. The aim of the method is to reduce the dimensionality of the data. The new variables, the principal components, are defined as *linear functions* of the original variables. If the first few principal components account for a large percentage of the variance of the observations (say above 70%), they can be used both to simplify subsequent analyses and to display and summarize the data in a parsimonious manner. See also **factor analysis**.

Principal components regression analysis: A procedure often used to overcome the problem of *multicollinearity* in regression, when simply deleting a number of the explanatory variables is not considered appropriate. Essentially, the response variable is regressed on a small number of principal component scores resulting from a *principal components analysis* of the explanatory variables.

Principal curves: Smooth one-dimensional curves that pass through the middle of a set of *multivariate data*, providing a non-linear summary of the data. The shape of such curves is suggested by the data.

Prior distributions: *Probability distributions* that summarize information about a *random variable* or parameter known or assumed at a given time point, *prior* to obtaining further information from empirical data. Used almost entirely within the context of *Bayesian inference*. In any particular study a variety of such distributions may be assumed. For example, *reference priors* represent minimal prior information; *clinical priors* are used to formalize opinion of well-informed specific individuals, often those taking part in the trial themselves. Finally, *sceptical priors* are used when large treatment differences are considered unlikely. See also **posterior distributions**.

Probability: The quantitative expression of the chance that an event will occur. Can be defined in a variety of ways, of which the most common is still that involving long term relative frequency, i.e.,

$$P(A) = \frac{\text{number of times } A \text{ occurs}}{\text{number of times } A \text{ could occur}}$$

For example, if out of 100 000 children born in a region, 51 000 are boys, then the probability of a boy is 0.51. See also **personal probability**.

Probability density: See **probability distribution**.

Probability distribution: For a discrete *random variable*, a mathematical formula that gives the probability of each value of the variable. See for example, *binomial distribution* and *Poisson distribution*. For a continuous random variable, a curve described by a mathematical formula which specifies, by way of areas under the curve, the probability that the variable falls within a particular interval. Examples include the *normal distribution* and the *exponential distribution*. In both cases the term *probability density* is also used. (A distinction is sometimes made between 'density' and 'distribution', when the latter is reserved for the probability that the random variable falls below some value. This distinction is not made in this dictionary; here probability distribution and probability density are used interchangeably.)

Probability-of-being-in-response function: A method for assessing the 'response experience' of a group of patients, by using a function of time, $P(t)$, which represents the probability of being 'in response' at time t. The purpose of such a function is to synthesize the different summary statistics commonly used to represent responses that are *binary variables*, namely, the proportion who respond and the average duration of response. The aim is to have a function which will highlight the distinction between a treatment that produces a high response rate but generally short-lived responses, and another that produces a low response rate but with longer response durations.

Probability paper: Graph paper structured in such a way that the values in the *cumulative frequency distribution* of a set of data from a *normal distribution* fall on a straight line. Can be used to assess sample data for normality.

Probability sample: A sample obtained by a method in which every individual in a *finite population* has a known (but not necessarily equal) chance of being included in the sample.

Proband: The clinically affected family member through whom attention is first drawn to a *pedigree* of particular interest to human genetics.

Probit analysis: A technique most commonly employed in bioassay, particularly toxicological experiments where sets of animals are subjected to known levels of a toxin, and a model is required to relate the proportion surviving at a particular dose, to the dose. In this type of analysis the *probit transformation* of a proportion is modelled as a *linear function* of the dose or, more commonly, the logarithm of the dose. Estimates of the parameters in the model are found by *maximum likelihood estimation*.

Probit transformation: A transformation, y, of a proportion, p, given by the equation

$$p = \frac{1}{\sqrt{2\pi}} \int_{-\infty}^{y} e^{-\frac{1}{2}u^2} \, du$$

The transformation is used in the analysis of *dose–response curves*. See also **probit analysis**.

Product limit estimator: A procedure for estimating the *survival function* for a set of *survival times*, some of which may be *censored observations*. The idea behind the procedure is that of the product of a number of conditional probabilities, so that, for example, the probability of a patient surviving two days after a liver transplant can be calculated as the probability of surviving one day, multiplied by the probability of surviving the second day given that the patient survived the first day. Specifically, the estimator is given by

$$\hat{S}(t) = \prod_{t_{(j)} \leq t} \left(1 - \frac{d_j}{r_j}\right)$$

where $\hat{S}(t)$ is the estimated survival function at time t, $t_{(1)} \leq t_{(2)} \cdots \leq t_{(n)}$ are the ordered survival times, r_j is the number of individuals at risk at time $t_{(j)}$ and d_j is the number of individuals who experience the event of

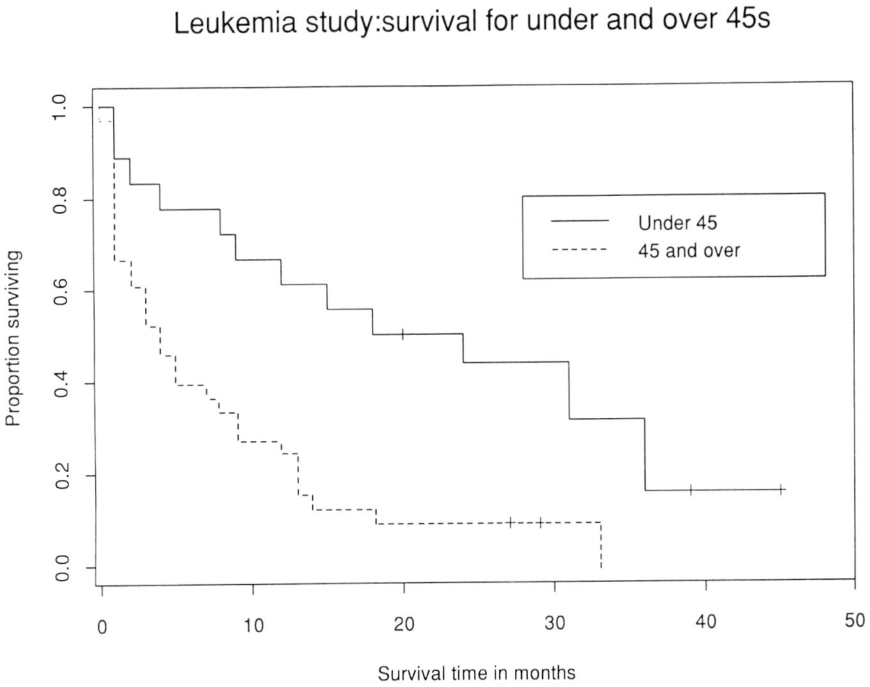

Fig 53 Survival curves estimated by the product limit estimator.

interest at time $t_{(j)}$. (Individuals censored at time $t_{(j)}$ are included in r_j). The resulting estimates form a step function that can be plotted to give a graphical display of survival experience. See also **Alshuler's estimator** and **Greenwood's formula**.

Profile analysis: A term sometimes used for the *analysis of variance* of *longitudinal data*.

Profile likelihood: See **likelihood**.

Prognostic scoring system: A method of combining the prognostic information contained in a number of *risk factors*, in a way which best predicts each patient's risk of disease. In many cases a *linear function* of scores is used, with the weights being derived from, for example, a *logistic regression*. An example of such a system, developed in the British Regional Heart Study for predicting men aged 40–59 years to be at risk of ischaemic heart disease over the next five years, is as follows:

51 × total serum cholesterol(mmol/l)
+ 5 × total time man has smoked(years)
+ 3 × systolic blood pressure(mmHg)

+ 100 if man has symptoms of angina
+ 170 if man can recall diagnosis of IHD
+ 50 if either parent died of heart trouble
+ 95 if man is diabetic

Prognostic variables: In medical investigations, an often used synonym for *explanatory variables.*

Programming: The act of planning and producing a set of instructions to solve a problem by computer. See also **algorithm**.

Progressively censored data: *Censored observations* that occur in *clinical trials* where the period of the study is fixed and patients enter the study at different times during that period. Since the entry times are not simultaneous, the censored times are also different. See also **singly censored data**.

Projection: The numerical outcome of a specific set of assumptions regarding future trends. See also **forecast**.

Projection plots: A general term for any technique that can be used to produce a graphical display of *multivariate data* by projecting the data into two dimensions, enabling a scatterplot to be drawn. Examples of such techniques are *principal components analysis, multidimensional scaling* and *projection pursuit.*

Projection pursuit: A procedure for obtaining a low-dimensional (usually two-dimensional) representation of *multivariate data*, that will be particularly useful in revealing interesting structure, such as the presence of distinct groups of observations. The low-dimensional representation is found by optimizing some pre-defined numerical criterion designed to reveal 'interesting' patterns.

Propensity score: A parameter that describes one aspect of the organization of a *clinical trial*, given by the *conditional probability* of assignment to a particular treatment, given a vector of values of concomitant variables.

Prophylactic trials: Synonym for **prevention trials**.

Proportional allocation: In *stratified random sampling*, the allocation of portions of the total sample to the individual *strata*, so that the sizes of these subsamples are proportional to the sizes of the corresponding strata.

Proportional hazards model: See **Cox's proportional hazards model**.

Proportional mortality rate: An index that may be used for comparing mortality rates for different diseases in different areas of a country or region or different time periods. The index is defined as

$$\text{PMR} = \frac{\text{disease deaths by region}}{\text{all deaths in region}} \Bigg/ \frac{\text{disease deaths in country}}{\text{all deaths in country}}$$

For example, the PMRs for motor neurone disease (MND) and Parkinson's disease (PD) (per 10 000) in a number of states of the USA are as follows:

State	MND	PD
California	28.37	25.85
Kansas	19.32	32.32
Vermont	11.93	25.84
Wyoming	18.46	18.46

Proportional-odds model: A model for investigating the dependence of an *ordinal variable* on a set of explanatory variables. In the most commonly employed version of the model, the cumulative probabilities, $P(y \leq k)$, where y is the response variable with categories $1 \leq 2 \leq 3 \cdots \leq c$, are modelled as *linear functions* of the explanatory variables via the *logistic transformation*, that is,

$$\log \frac{P(y \leq k)}{1 - P(y \leq k)} = \beta_0 + \beta_1 x_1 \cdots + \beta_q x_q$$

The name proportional-odds arises since the *odds ratio* of having a score of k or less for two different sets of values of the explanatory variables does not depend on k.

Prospective study: Studies in which individuals are followed up over a period of time. A common example of this type of investigation is where samples of individuals exposed and not exposed to a possible *risk factor* for a particular disease are followed forward in time, to determine what happens to them with respect to the illness under investigation. At the end of a suitable time period a comparison of the *incidence* of the disease amongst the exposed and non-exposed is made. A classic example of such a study is that undertaken amongst British doctors in the 1950s, to investigate the relationship between smoking and death from lung cancer. See also **retrospective study** and **cohort study**.

Protective efficacy of a vaccine: The proportion of cases of disease prevented by the vaccine, usually estimated as

$$\text{PE} = (\text{ARU} - \text{ARV})/\text{ARU}$$

where ARV and ARU are the *attack rates* of the disease under study amongst the vaccinated and unvaccinated cohorts, respectively. For example, if the rate of the disease is 100 per 10 000 in an unvaccinated group but only 30 per 10 000 in a comparable vaccinated group, the PE is 70%. Essentially equivalent to *attributable risk*.

Protocol: A formal document outlining the proposed procedures for carrying out a *clinical trial*. The main features of the document are study objectives, patient selection criteria, treatment schedules, methods of patient evaluation, trial design, procedures for dealing with *protocol violations* and plans for statistical analysis.

Protocol violations: Patients who either deliberately or accidentally have not followed one or other aspect of the *protocol* for carrying out a *clinical trial*. For example, they may not have taken their prescribed medication. Such patients are said to show *non-compliance*.

Proximity matrix: A general term for either *similarity matrices* or *dissimilarity matrices*. In general such matrices are symmetric, but *asymmetric proximity matrices* do occur in some situations.

Pseudorandom numbers: A sequence of numbers generated by a specific computer *algorithm*, which satisfy particular statistical tests of randomness. So although not random, the numbers appear so.

Pseudo R^2: An index sometimes used in assessing the fit of specific types of models, particularly those for modelling *survival times*. It is defined as

$$1 - \frac{\ln L(\text{present model})}{\ln L(\text{model without covariates})}$$

where L represents *likelihood*. Expresses the relative decrease of the *log-likelihood* of the present model as opposed to the model without covariates.

Publication bias: The possible bias in published accounts of, for example, *clinical trials*, produced by editors of journals being more likely to accept a paper if a statistically significant effect has been demonstrated. See also **funnel plot**.

Pulse data: A series of measurements of the concentration of a hormone, or other blood constituent, in blood samples taken from a single organism at regular time intervals. See also **episodic hormone data**.

P-value: The probability of the observed data (or data showing a more extreme departure from the *null hypothesis*) when the null hypothesis is true. See also **misinterpretation of P-values**, **significance test** and **significance level**.

Q

QOL: Acronym for **quality-of-life data**.

Q–Q plot: Synonym for **quantile–quantile plot**.

Q-techniques: The class of data analysis methods that look for relationships between the individuals in a set of *multivariate data*. Includes *cluster analysis* and *multidimensional scaling*, although the term is most commonly used for a type of *factor analysis* applied to an $n \times n$ matrix of 'correlations' between individuals rather than between variables. See also **R-techniques**.

Quadrant sampling: A sampling procedure used with *spatial data* in which sample areas (the quadrants) are taken, and the number of objects or events of interest occurring in each recorded.

Quadratic discriminant function: See **discriminant analysis**.

Quadratic function: A function of the form

$$Q = \sum_{i=1}^{n} \sum_{j=1}^{n} a_{ij} x_i x_j$$

important in *multivariate analysis* and *analysis of variance*.

Quality-adjusted survival times: The weighted sum of different time episodes making up a patient's *survival time*, with the weights reflecting the *quality-of-life* of each period.

Quality assurance: Any procedure or method for collecting, processing or analysing data that is aimed at maintaining or improving the *reliability* or *validity* of the data.

Quality control angle chart: A modified version of the *cusum*, derived by representing each value, taken in order, by a line of some unit length in a direction proportional to its value. The line for each successive value starts at the end of the preceeding line. A change in direction on the chart indicates a change in the mean value. Often referred to as a *quangle*.

Quality control procedures: Statistical procedures designed to ensure that the precision and accuracy of, for example, a laboratory test, are maintained within acceptable limits. The simplest such procedure involves a chart (usually called a *control chart*) with three horizontal lines, one drawn at the target level of the relevant *control statistic*, and the others, called *action lines*, drawn at some prespecified distance above and below the target level. The process is judged to be at an *acceptable quality level* as long as the observed control statistic lies between the two lines, and to be at a *rejectable quality level* if either of these lines are crossed.

Quality-of-life (QOL) variables: A broad range of variables describing a patient's subjective reactions to and perceptions of his or her environment. See also **Barthel index**.

Quangle: See **quality control angle chart**.

Quantal assay: An experiment in which groups of subjects are exposed to different doses of, usually, a drug, to which a particular number respond. Data from such assays are often analysed using the *probit transformation*, and interest generally centres on estimating the *median effective dose* or *lethal dose 50*.

Quantal variable: Synonym for **binary variable**.

Quantile–quantile (Q–Q) plot: An informal method for assessing assumptions when fitting statistical models or using significance tests. For example, for investigating the assumption that a set of data is from a *normal distribution*, the ordered sample values, $x_{(1)}, x_{(2)}, \ldots x_{(n)}$, are plotted against the values

$$\Phi^{-1}(p_i)$$

where $p_i = i - \frac{1}{2}$ and

$$\Phi(x) = \int_{-\infty}^{x} \frac{1}{\sqrt{2\pi}} e^{-\frac{1}{2}u^2} du$$

(This is usually known as a *normal probability plot*). Departures from normality are indicated by departures from linearity in the plot. (See Fig. 54 opposite.) See also **chi-squared probability plot**.

Quantiles: Divisions of a *probability distribution* or *frequency distribution* into equal, ordered subgroups, for example, *quartiles* or *percentiles*.

Quantit model: A three-parameter non-linear *logistic regression model*.

Quartiles: The values that divide a *frequency distribution* or *probability distribution* into four equal parts.

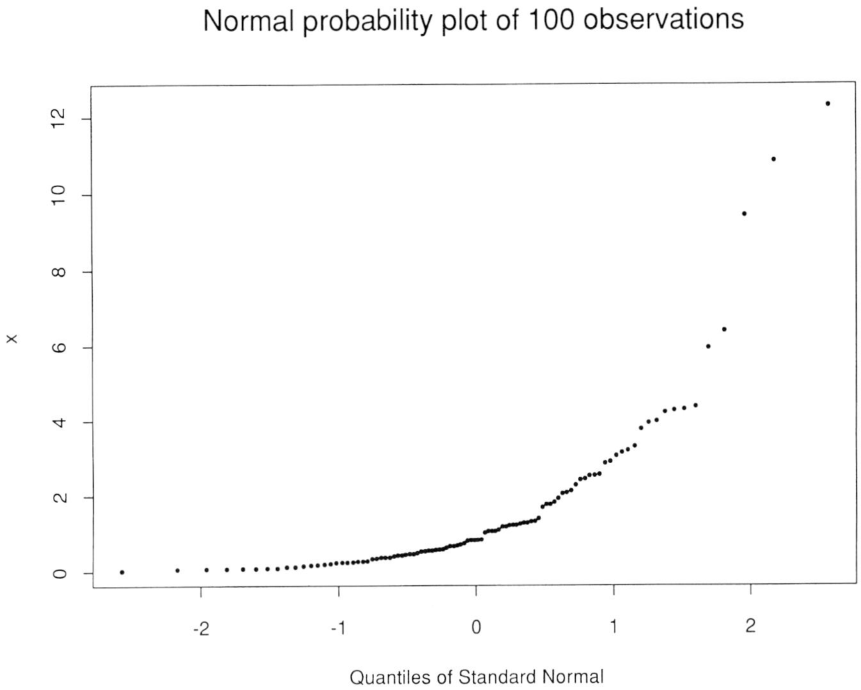

Fig 54 An example of a quantile–quantile plot.

Quasi-experiment: A term used for studies that resemble experiments but are weak on some of the characteristics, particularly that manipulation of subjects to groups is not under the investigator's control. For example, if interest centred on the health effects of a natural disaster, those who experience the disaster can be compared with those who do not, but subjects cannot be deliberately assigned (randomly or not) to the two groups. See also **prospective studies, experimental design** and **clinical trials**.

Quasi-independence: A form of independence for a *contingency table*, conditional on restricting attention to a particular part of the table only. For example, in the following table showing the social class of sons and their fathers, it might be of interest to assess whether, once a son has moved out of his father's class, his destination class is independent of that of his father. This would entail testing whether independence holds in the table after ignoring the entries in the main diagonal.

Father's	**Son's social class**		
social class	Upper	Middle	Lower
Upper	588	395	159
Middle	349	714	447
Lower	114	320	411

Quasi-likelihood: A function that is used as the basis for the estimation of parameters where it is not possible (and/or desirable) to make a particular distributional assumption about the observations, with the consequence that it is not possible to write down their *likelihood*. The function depends on the assumed relationship between the mean and the variance of the observations.

Quetelet's index: A measure of obesity given by weight divided by the square of the height.

Queuing theory: A largely mathematical theory concerned with the study of various factors relating to queues, such as the distribution of arrivals, the average time spent in the queue, etc. Used in medical investigations of waiting times for hospital beds, for example.

Quick and dirty methods: A term once applied to many *distribution-free methods*, presumably to highlight their general ease of computation and their imagined inferiority to the corresponding parametric procedure.

Quintiles: The set of four variate values that divide a *frequency distribution* or a *probability distribution* into five equal parts.

Quitting ill effect: A problem that occurs most often in studies of smoker cessation, where smokers frequently quit smoking following the onset of disease symptoms or the diagnosis of a life-threatening disease, thereby creating an anomalous rise in, for example, lung cancer risk following smoking cessation relative to continuing smokers. Such an increase has been reported in many studies.

Quota sample: A sample in which the units are not selected completely at random, but in terms of a certain number of units in each of a number of categories; for example, 10 men over age 40, 25 women between ages 30 and 35. Widely used in opinion polls. See also **sample survey** and **random sample**.

R

Radial plot of odds ratios: A diagram used to display the *odds ratios* calculated from a number of different *clinical trials* of the same treatment(s). Often useful in a *meta-analysis* of the results. The diagram consists of a plot of $y = \hat{\triangle}/SE(\hat{\triangle})$ against $x = 1/SE(\hat{\triangle})$, where $\hat{\triangle}$ is the logarithm of the odds ratio from a particular study. An example of such a plot is shown overleaf. Some features of this display are:

- every estimate has unit standard error in the y direction. The y scale is drawn as a ± 2 error bar to indicate this explicitly;
- the numerical value of an odds ratio can be read off by extrapolating a line from (0,0) through (x, y) to the circular scale drawn, the horizontal line corresponds to an odds ratio of unity. Also, approximate 95% confidence limits can be read off by extrapolating lines from (0,0) through $(x, y+2), (x, y-2)$ respectively;
- points with large $SE(\hat{\triangle})$ fall near the origin, while points with small $SE(\hat{\triangle})$, that is, the more informative estimates, fall well away from the origin and naturally look more informative.

Rand coefficient: An index for assessing the similarity of alternative classifications of the same set of observations. Used most often when comparing the solutions from two methods of *cluster analysis* applied to the same set of data. The coefficient is given by

$$R = \left[T - 0.5P - 0.5Q + \binom{n}{2}\right] \Big/ \binom{n}{2}$$

where

$$T = \sum_{i=1}^{g} \sum_{j=1}^{g} m_{ij}^2 - n$$

$$P = \sum_{i=1}^{g} m_{i.}^2 - n$$

$$Q = \sum_{j=1}^{g} m_{.j}^2 - n$$

The quantity m_{ij} is the number of individuals in common between the ith cluster of the first solution and the jth cluster of the second (the clusters in the two solutions may each be labelled arbitrarily from 1 to g, where g

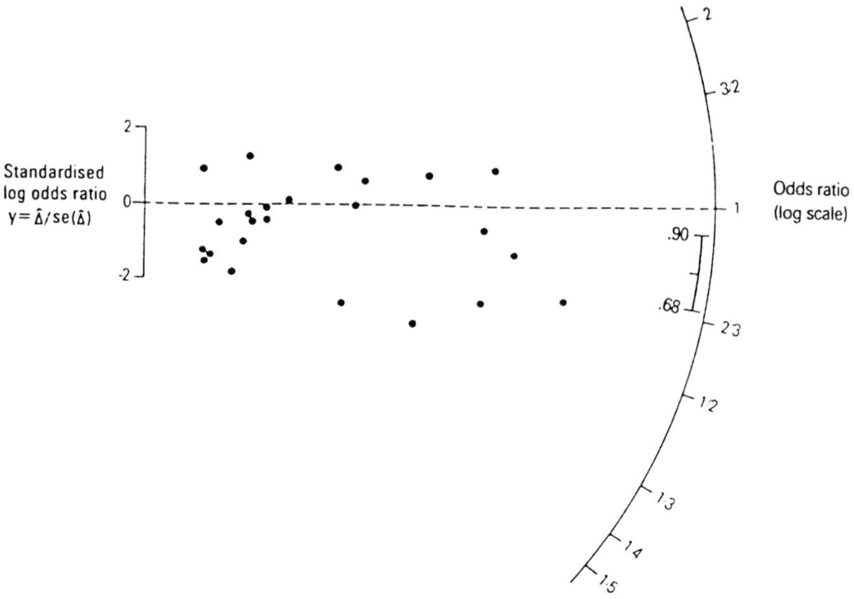

Fig 55 Radial plot of odds ratios.

is the number of clusters). The terms $m_{i.}$ and $m_{.j}$ are appropriate marginal totals of the matrix of m_{ij} values, and n is the number of observations. The coefficient lies in the interval (0,1) and takes its upper limit only when there is complete agreement between the two classifications.

Random: Governed by chance; not completely determined by other factors. Non-deterministic.

Random allocation: A method for forming treatment and control groups, particularly in the context of a *clinical trial*. Subjects receive the active treatment or placebo on the basis of the outcome of a chance event, for example, tossing a coin. The method provides an impartial procedure for allocation of treatments to individuals, free from personal biases, and ensures a firm footing for the application of significance tests and most of the rest of the statistical methodology likely to be used. Additionally, the method distributes the effects of *concomitant variables*, both observed and unobserved, in a statistically acceptable fashion. See also **block randomization**, **minimization** and **biased coin method**.

Random effects: The effects attributable to a (usually) infinite set of levels of a factor, of which only a *random sample* occur in the data. For example, the investigator may be interested in the effects of a particular class of drug on a response variable, and uses a random sample of drugs from the class in a study. *Random effects models* arise when all the factors in the investigation are of this kind. See also **fixed effects**.

Random effects model: See **random effects**.

Randomization tests: Procedures for determining statistical significance directly from data, without recourse to some particular *sampling distribution*. The data are divided (permuted) repeatedly between treatments, and for each division (permutation) the relevant *test statistic* (for example, a t or F), is calculated to determine the proportion of the data permutations that provide as large a test statistic as that associated with the observed data. If that proportion is smaller than some significance level α, the results are significant at the α level.

Randomized block design (RBD): An experimental design in which the treatments in each *block* are assigned to the experimental units in random order.

Randomized clinical trial (RCT): A *clinical trial* that involves formation of treatment groups by the process of *random allocation*.

Randomized consent design: A design originally introduced to overcome some of the perceived ethical problems facing clinicians entering patients in *randomized clinical trials*. After the patient's eligibility is established, the patient is randomised to one of two treatments A and B. Patients randomised to A are approached for patient consent. They are asked if they are willing to receive therapy A for their illness. All potential risks, benefits and treatment options are discussed. If the patient agrees, treatment A is given. If not, the patient receives treatment B or some other alternative treatment. Those patients randomly assigned to group B are similarly asked about treatment B, and transferred to an alternative treatment if consent is not given. See also **Zelen's single-consent design**.

Randomized response technique: A procedure for collecting information on sensitive issues by means of a survey, in which an element of chance is introduced as to what question a respondent has to answer. In a survey about abortion, for example, a woman might be posed both the questions 'have you had an abortion' and 'have you never had an abortion', and instructed to respond to one or the other depending on the outcome of a randomizing device under her control. The response is now not revealing since no one except the respondent is aware of which question has been answered. Nevertheless, the data obtained can be used to estimate quantities of interest, here, for example, the proportion of women who have had an abortion (π), if the probability of selecting the question 'have you had an abortion', P, is known and is not equal to 0.5. If y is the proportion of 'yes' answers to this question in a *random sample* of n respondents, one estimator of π is given by

$$\hat{\pi} = \frac{y - (1 - P)}{2P - 1}$$

This estimator is *unbiased* and has variance, V:

$$V = \frac{\pi(1 - \pi)}{n} + \frac{P(1 - P)}{n(2P - 1)}$$

Random model: One containing random or probabilistic elements. See also **deterministic model**.

Random sample: Either a set of n independent and identically distributed *random variables*, or a sample of n individuals selected from a population in such a way that each sample of the same size is equally likely.

Random variable: A variable, the values of which occur according to some specified *probability distribution*.

Random variation: The variation in a data set unexplained by identifiable sources.

Random walk: The motion of a 'particle' that moves in discrete jumps with certain probabilities from point to point. At its simplest, the particle would start at the point $x = k$ on the x axis at time $t = 0$, and at each subsequent time, $t = 1, 2, \cdots$, it moves one step to the right or left with probabilities p and $1 - p$ respectively. As a concrete example, the position of the particle might represent the size of a population of individuals, and a step to the left corresponds to a death and to the right a birth. Here the process would stop if the particle ever reached the origin, $x = 0$, which is consequently termed an *absorbing barrier*.

Range: The difference between the largest and smallest observations in a data set. Often used as an easy-to-calculate measure of the *dispersion* in a set of observations, but not recommended for this task because of its sensitivity to *outliers*.

Range of equivalence: The range of differences between two treatments being compared in a *clinical trial*, within which it is not possible to make a definite choice of treatment. For example, if the true treatment difference is summarized by a parameter, δ, with large values of δ corresponding to superiority of the new treatment, there may be a certain threshold level, δ_L, that the new treatment must achieve before it can be considered, with values of $\delta < \delta_L$ being regarded as not providing sufficient evidence in favour of the new treatment. Another value, δ_U, may also be postulated, where only values of δ such that $\delta > \delta_U$ provide evidence of the clinical superiority of the new treatment. The interval, (δ_L, δ_U) is the range of equivalence of the two treatments.

Rank adjacency statistic: A statistic used to summarize *autocorrelations* of *spatial data*. Given by

$$D = \sum\sum w_{ij}|y_i - y_j| / \sum\sum w_{ij}$$

where $y_i = \text{rank}(x_i)$, x_i is the data value for location i, and the w_{ij} are a set of weights representing some function of distance or contact between regions i and j. The simplest weighting option is to define

$$\begin{aligned} w_{ij} &= 1 \quad \text{if regions } i \text{ and } j \text{ are adjacent} \\ &= 0 \quad \text{otherwise} \end{aligned}$$

in which case D becomes the average absolute rank difference over all pairs of adjacent regions.The theoretical distribution of D is not known, but spatial clustering (or positive spatial autocorrelation) in the data will be reflected by the tendency for adjacent data values to have similar ranks, so that the value of D will tend to be smaller than otherwise. See also **Moran's *I***.

Rank correlation coefficients: Correlation coefficients that depend only on the ranks of the variables, not on their observed values. Examples include *Kendall's tau statistics* and *Spearman's rho*.

Ranking: The process of sorting a set of variable values into either ascending or descending order.

Rank of a matrix: The number of linearly independent rows or columns of a matrix of numbers.

Rank order statistics: Statistics based only on the ranks of the sample observations, for example *Kendall's tau statistics*.

Ranks: The relative positions of the members of a sample with respect to some characteristic.

Rasch model: A model often used in the theory of cognitive tests. The model proposes that the probability that an examinee i with ability quantified by a parameter, δ_i, answers item j correctly is given by

$$P(x_{ij} = 1|\delta_i, \epsilon_j) = \delta_i\epsilon_j/(1 + \delta_i\epsilon_j)$$

where ϵ_j is a measure of the simplicity of the item. This probability is commonly rewritten in the form

$$P(x_{ij} = 1|\theta_i, \sigma_j) = \frac{\exp(\theta_i - \sigma_j)}{1 + \exp(\theta_i - \sigma_j)}$$

where $\exp(\theta_i) = \delta_i$ and $\exp(-\sigma_j) = \epsilon_j$. In this version, θ_i is still called the *ability parameter*, but σ_j is now termed the *item difficulty*.

Ratchet scan statistic: A statistic used in investigations attempting to detect a relatively sharp increase in disease incidence for a season, superimposed on a constant incidence over the entire year. If $n_1, n_2, \cdots, n_{12}$ are the total number of observations in January, February, $\cdots$, December, respectively (months are assumed to be of equal lengths), then the sum of k consecutive months starting with month i can be written as

$$S_i^k = \sum_{j=1}^{(i+k-1)\text{mod}12} n_j$$

The ratchet scan statistic is based on the maximum number falling within k consecutive months, and is defined as

$$T^k = \max_{i=1,\cdots,12} S_i^k$$

Under the hypothesis of a *uniform distribution* of events, i.e., the *expected value* of n_i is $N/12$ for all $i = 1, 2, \cdots, 12$, where N = the total number of events in the year, it can be shown that

$$P(T^k \geq n) = \sum \frac{N!}{12^N \prod_{i=1}^{12} n_i!}$$

where the sum is taken over all the values of $(n_1, n_2, \cdots, n_{12})$ that yield $T^k \geq n$. Approximations for the distribution for $k = 1$ have been derived, but not for $k > 1$.

Rate: A measure of the frequency of some phenomenon of interest, given by

$$\text{Rate} = \frac{\text{number of events in specified period}}{\text{average population during the period}}$$

(The resulting value is often multiplied by some power of ten to convert it to a whole number.)

Ratio variable: A *continuous variable* that has a fixed rather than an arbitrary zero point. Examples are height, weight and temperature measured in degrees Kelvin. See also **categorical variable** and **ordinal variable**.

RBD: Abbreviation for **randomized block design**.

RCT: Abbreviation for **randomized clinical trial**.

Recall bias: A possible source of *bias*, particularly in a *retrospective study*, caused by differential recall amongst cases and controls, in general by under reporting of exposure in the control group. See also **ascertainment bias**.

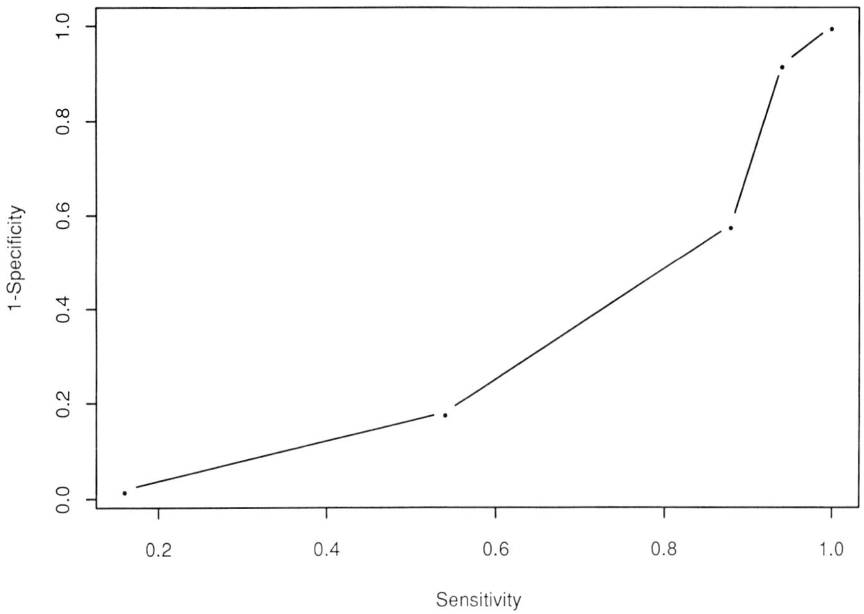

Fig 56 An example of an ROC curve.

Receiver operating characteristic (ROC) curves: A plot of the *sensitivity* of a *diagnostic test* against one minus its *specificity*, as the cutoff criterion for indicating a positive test is varied. Often used in choosing between competing tests, although the procedure takes no account of the *prevalence* of the disease being tested for. As an example, consider the following ratings from 1 (definitely normal) to 5 (definitely diseased) arising from 50 normal and 50 diseased subjects.

	1	2	3	4	5	**Total**
Normal	4	17	20	8	1	50
Diseased	3	3	17	19	8	50

If the rating of 5 is used as the cutoff for identifying diseased cases, then the sensitivity is estimated as $8/50 = 0.16$, and the specificity as $49/50 = 0.98$. Now, using the rating 4 as cutoff leads to a sensitivity of $27/50 = 0.54$ and a specificity of $41/50 = 0.82$. The values of (sensitivity, 1-specificity) as the cutoff decreases from 5 to 1 are (0.16, 0.02), (0.54, 0.18), (0.88, 0.58), (0.94, 0.92), (1.00, 1.00). These points are plotted in the diagram shown. This is the required receiver operating characteristic curve.

Reciprocal transformation: A transformation of the form $y = 1/x$, which is particularly useful for certain types of variables. Resistances, for example, become conductances, and times become speeds. In some cases the transformation can lead to linear relationships, for example, airways resistance against lung volume is non-linear, but airways conductance against lung volume is linear.

Recombination frequency: The number of recombinants divided by the total number of progeny. This frequency is used as a guide in assessing the relative distances between loci on a genetic map.

Record linkage: A method for assembling the information contained in two or more records on a patient that insures that the same individual is counted only once.

Rectangular distribution: Synonym for **uniform distribution**.

Recurrence risk: The probability of disease for an individual given that a relative is diseased.

Recursive: A function or sequence is defined recursively if

- the value of $f(0)$ and
- the value of $f(n+1)$, given the value of $f(n)$, are both stated.
  For example, the factorial function may be defined by
- $f(0) = 1$,
- $f(n+1) = nf(n)$ for $n = 0, 1, 2, \cdots$.

Reference interval: A range of values for a variable that encompasses the values obtained from the majority of normal subjects. Often used as the basis for assessing the results of *diagnostic tests* in the classification of individuals as normal or abnormal with respect to a particular variable.

Reference population: The standard against which a population that is being studied can be compared.

Reference priors: See **prior distributions**.

Regression analysis: A general term for methods of analysis that are concerned with estimating the parameters in some postulated relationship between a response variable and one or more explanatory variables. Particular examples are *linear regression*, *logistic regression* and *multiple regression*.

Regression coefficient: See **multiple regression**.

Regression diagnostics: Procedures designed to investigate the assumptions underlying a *regression analysis*, for example, normality, homogeneity of variance; or to examine the *influence* of particular data points or small groups of data points on the estimated *regression coefficients*. See also **residuals**, **Cook's distance** and **influence**.

Regression dilution: The term applied when a covariate in a model can only be measured with error. In general, if the model is correctly specified in terms of the 'true' covariate, then a similar form of the model with a simple error structure will not hold for the observed values. In such cases, ignoring the measurement error will lead to biased estimates of the parameters in the model. Often also refered to as the *errors-in-variables problem*. See also **attenuation, latent variables** and **structural equation modelling**.

Regression through the origin: In some situations a relationship between two variables estimated by *regression analysis* is expected to pass through the origin, because the true mean of the dependent variable is known to be zero when the value of the explanatory variable is zero. In such situations the *linear regression* model is forced to pass through the origin by setting the intercept parameter to zero and estimating only the slope parameter.

Regression to the mean: The process first noted by Sir Francis Galton that 'each peculiarity in man is shared by his kinsmen, but on the average to a less degree.' Hence the tendency, for example, for tall parents to produce tall offspring but who, on average, are shorter than their parents. The term is now generally used to label the phenomenon that a variable that is extreme on its first measurement will tend to be closer to the centre of the distribution for a later measurement. For example, in a screening program for hypertension, only persons with high blood pressure are asked to return for a second measure. On the average, the second measure taken will be less than the first.

Regression weight: Synonym for **regression coefficient**.

Reification: The process of naming *latent variables* and the consequent discussion of such things as quality of life and racial prejudice as though they were physical quantities in the same sense as, for example, are length and weight.

Rejectable quality level: See **quality control procedures**.

Relative efficiency: The ratio of the variances of two possible estimates of a parameter, or the ratio of the sample sizes required by two statistical procedures to achieve the same *power*.

Relative risk: A measure of the association between exposure to a particular factor and risk of a certain outcome, calculated as

$$\text{relative risk} = \frac{\text{incidence rate among exposed}}{\text{incidence rate among nonexposed}}$$

Thus a relative risk of 5, for example, means that an exposed person is 5 times as likely to have the disease than one who is not exposed. Relative risk does **not** measure the probability that someone with the factor will develop the disease. The disease may be rare amongst both the nonexposed and the exposed. See also **incidence** and **attributable risk**.

Relative standardized mortality rate: The ratio of the *standardized mortality rate* for a particular cause of death, divided by the all-causes SMR. This index attempts to make an adjustment for overall differences in mortality due to *healthy worker effects* or other differences between the study and referant populations.

Relative survival: The ratio of the observed survival of a given group of patients to the survival the group would have experienced based on the *life table* of the population from which they were diagnosed.

Release targets: A term used in the pharmaceutical industry for in-house limits for the average potency of a batch of some drug. These limits are calculated to give some degree of assurance that the average potency of a batch released is within the limits demanded by a regulatory body such as the *Food and Drug Administration*. Customarily used limits are

$$(L + 1.645\hat{\sigma} + \hat{s}, U - 1.645\hat{\sigma})$$

where $\hat{s}$ is the estimated stability loss in potency over the expiration period and $\hat{\sigma}$ is the estimated variablity of the assay determining potency. The terms U and L are the upper and lower limits on potency set by the regulatory body.

Reliability: The extent to which the same measurements of individuals obtained under different conditions yield similar results. See also **intraclass correlation** and **kappa coefficient**.

REML: Acronym for **restricted maximum likelihood estimation**.

Repeatability: The closeness of the results obtained in the same test material by the same observer or technician using the same equipment, apparatus and/or reagents over reasonably short intervals of time.

Repeated measures data: See **longitudinal data**.

Replicate observation: An independent observation obtained under conditions as nearly identical to the original as the nature of the investigation will permit.

Reproducibility: The closeness of results obtained on the same test material under changes of reagents, conditions, technicians, apparatus, laboratories and so on.

Reproduction rate: See **basic reproduction rate**.

Research hypothesis: Synonym for **alternative hypothesis**.

Residual: The difference between the observed value of a response variable (y_i) and the value predicted by some model of interest ($\hat{y}_i$). Examination of a set of residuals, usually by informal graphical techniques, allows the assumptions made in the model fitting exercise, for example, normality, homogeneity of variance, to be checked. Generally, discrepant observations have large residuals, but some form of standardization may be necessary in many situations to allow identification of patterns amongst the residuals that may be a cause for concern. The usual *standardized residual* for observation y_i is calculated from

$$\frac{y_i - \hat{y}_i}{s\sqrt{1 - h_i}}$$

where s^2 is the estimated residual variance after fitting the model of interest, and h_i is the ith diagonal element of the *hat matrix*. An alternative definition of a standardized residual (sometimes known as the *Studentized residual*), is

$$\frac{y_i - \hat{y}_i}{s_{(-i)}\sqrt{1 - h_i}}$$

where now $s^2_{(-i)}$ is the estimated residual variance from fitting the model after the exclusion of the ith observation. See also **regression diagnostics, Cook's distance** and **influence**.

Residual sum of squares: See **analysis of variance**.

Response bias: The systematic component of the difference between information provided by survey respondent and the 'truth'.

Response feature analysis: An approach to the analysis of *longitudinal data* involving the calculation of suitable summary measures from the set of repeated measures on each subject. For example, the mean of the subject's measurements might be calculated, or the maximum value of the response variable over the repeated measurements. Simple methods such as *Student's t-tests* or *Mann–Whitney tests* are then applied to these summary measures to assess differences between treatments.

Response rate: The proportion of subjects who respond to, usually, a postal questionnaire.

Response variable: The variable of primary importance in medical investigations, since the major objective is usually to study the effects of treatment and/or other explanatory variables on this variable, and to provide suitable models for the relationship between it and the explanatory variables.

Restricted likelihood: See **likelihood**.

Restricted maximum likelihood estimation (REML): A method of estimation in which estimators of parameters are derived by maximizing the *restricted likelihood* rather than the *likelihood* itself. Most often used for estimating *variance components* in a *generalized linear model.*

Responders versus non-responders analysis: A comparison of the survival experience of patients according to whether or not there is some observed response to treatment. In general such analyses are invalid because the groups are defined by a factor not known at the start of treatment.

Resubstitution error rate: The estimate of the proportion of subjects misclassified by a rule derived from a *discriminant analysis*, obtained by reclassifying the *training set* using the rule. As an estimate of likely future performance of the rule, it is almost always optimistic, i.e., it will underestimate the 'true' misclassification rate. See also **jackknife**.

Retrospective cohort study: See **retrospective study**.

Retrospective study: A general term for studies in which all the events of interest occur prior to the onset of the study, and findings are based on looking backward in time. Most common is the *case–control study*, in which comparisons are made between individuals who have a particular disease or condition (the cases) and individuals who do not have the disease (the controls). A sample of cases is selected from the population of individuals who have the disease of interest, and a sample of controls is taken from amongst those individuals known not to have the disease. Information about possible *risk factors* for the disease is then obtained retrospectively for each person in the study by examining past records, by interviewing each person and/or interviewing their relatives, or in some other way. In order to make the cases and controls otherwise comparable, they are frequently matched on characteristics known to be strongly related to both disease and exposure, leading to a *matched case–control study*. Age, sex and socioeconomic status are examples of commonly used matching variables. Also commonly encountered is the *retrospective cohort study*, in which a past cohort of individuals are identified from previous information, for example, employment records, and their subsequent mortality or morbidity determined and compared with the corresponding experience of some suitable control group.

Ridge regression: A method of *regression analysis* designed to overcome the possible problem of *multicollinearity* among the explanatory variables. Such multicollinearity makes it difficult to estimate the separate effects of variables on the response. By allowing regression estimates to be biased, this form of regression results in increased precision.

Ridit analysis: A method of analysis for *ordinal variables* that proceeds from the assumption that the ordered categorical scale is an approximation to an underlying, but not directly measurable, continuous variable. The successive categories are assumed to correspond to consecutive intervals on the underlying continuum. Numerical values called ridits are calculated for each category, these values being estimates of the probability that a subject's value on the underlying variable is less than or equal to the midpoint of the corresponding interval. These scores are then used in subsequent analyses involving the variable.

Risk: A term often used in medicine for the probability that an event will occur, for example, that a person will become ill or will die.

Risk factor: An aspect of personal behaviour or lifestyle, an environmental exposure, or an inborn or inherited characteristic, which is thought to be associated with a particular disease or condition.

Risk set: A term used in *survival analysis* for those individuals who are alive and uncensored at a time just prior to some particular time point.

Robust estimation: Methods of estimation that work well, not only under ideal conditions, but also under conditions representing a departure from an assumed distribution or model. See also **high breakdown methods**.

Robust regression: A general class of statistical procedures designed to reduce the sensitivity of the parameter estimates to failures in the assumption of the model. For example, *least squares estimation* is known to be sensitive to *outliers*, but the impact of such observations can be reduced by basing the estimation process not on a sum-of-squares criterion, but on a sum of absolute values criterion.

Robust statistics: Statistical procedures and tests that still work reasonably well even when the assumptions on which they are based are mildly (or perhaps moderately) violated. *Student's t-test*, for example, is robust against departures from normality. See also **high breakdown methods**.

ROC curves: Abbreviation for **receiver operating characteristic curves**.

Rootogram: A diagram obtained from a histogram in which the rectangles represent the square roots of the observed frequencies rather than the frequencies themselves. The idea behind such a diagram is to remove the tendency for the variability of a count to increase with its typical size. See also **hanging rootogram**.

Rosenbaum's test: A *distribution-free method* for the equality of the scale parameters of two populations known to have the same median. The *test statistic* is the total number of values in the sample from the first population that are either smaller than the smallest or larger than the largest values in the sample from the second population.

Rosenthal effect: The observation that investigators often find what they expect to find from a study. For example, in a reliability study in which auscultatory measurements of the foetal heart rate were compared with the electronically recorded rate, it was found that when the true rate was under 130 beats per minute the hospital staff tended to overestimate it, and when it was over 150 they tended to underestimate it.

Rounding: The procedure used for reporting numerical information to fewer decimal places than used during analysis. The rule generally adopted is that excess digits are simply discarded if the first of them is less than five, otherwise the last retained digit is increased by one. So rounding 127.249 341 to three decimal places gives 127.249.

Round robin study: A term sometimes used for interlaboratory comparisons in which samples of a material manufactured to well-defined specifications are sent out to the participating laboratories for analysis. The results are used to assess differences between laboratories and to identify possible sources of incompatability or other anomalies. See also **interlaboratory trials**.

Roy's largest root criterion: See **multivariate analysis of variance**.

R-techniques: The class of data analysis methods that look for relationships between the variables in a set of *multivariate data*. Includes *principal components analysis* and *factor analysis*. See also **Q-techniques**.

Rugplot: A method of displaying graphically a sample of values on a continuous variable by indicating their positions on a horizontal line.

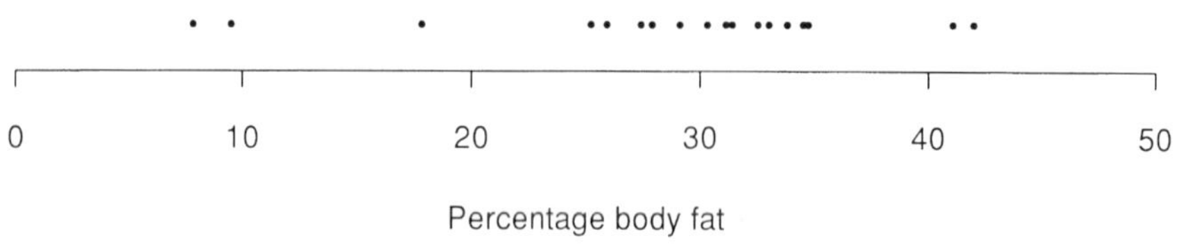

Fig 57 A rugplot of percentage body fat in a number of individuals.

Rule of threes: A rule which states that if in n trials, zero events of interest are observed, a 95% confidence bound on the underlying rate is $3/n$.

Run-in: A period of observation, prior to the formation of treatment groups by *random allocation*, during which subjects acquire experience with the major components of a study *protocol*. Those subjects who experience difficulty complying with the protocol are excluded, while the group of proven compliers are randomized into the trial. The rationale behind such a procedure is that, in general, a study with higher compliance will have higher *power* because the observed effects of the difference between treatment groups will not be subjected to the diluting effects of non-compliance.

Runs: In a series of observations, the occurrence of an uninterrupted sequence of the same value. For example, in the series

111224333333

there are four 'runs', the single value, 4, being regarded as a run of length unity.

Runs test: A test frequently used to detect *serial correlations*. The test consists of counting the number of *runs*, or sequences of positive and negative residuals, and comparing the result with the *expected value* under the *null hypothesis* of independence. If the sample observations consist of n_1 positive and n_2 negative residuals, with both n_1 and n_2 greater than 10, the distribution of the length of runs can be approximated by a *normal distribution* with mean, μ, and variance, σ^2, given by

$$\mu = \frac{2n_1n_2}{n_1 + n_2} + 1$$
$$\sigma^2 = \frac{2n_1n_2(2n_1n_2 - n_1 - n_2)}{(n_1 + n_2)^2(n_1 + n_2 - 1)}$$

Rvachev–Baroyan–Longini model: A space–time predictive model of the spread of influenza epidemics. The model contains two parameters, the *contact rate*, which is the number of people with whom an infectious individual will make contact daily sufficient to pass infection, and the *infectious period*.

RV-coefficient: A measure of the similarity of two configurations of n data points, given by

$$\mathrm{RV}(\mathbf{X}, \mathbf{Y}) = \frac{\mathrm{tr}(\mathbf{XY}'\mathbf{YX}')}{\{\mathrm{tr}(\mathbf{XX}')^2\mathrm{tr}(\mathbf{YY}')^2\}^{\frac{1}{2}}}$$

where $\mathbf{X}$ and $\mathbf{Y}$ are the matrices describing the two configurations. Several techniques of *multivariate analysis* can be expressed in terms of maximizing $\mathrm{RV}(\mathbf{X}, \mathbf{Y})$ for some definition of $\mathbf{X}$ and $\mathbf{Y}$.

S

Saddle point approximations: Techniques for the asymptotic evaluation of integrals of the form

$$I_n = \int f(t) e^{-ng(t)} \mathrm{d}t$$

in the limit for large n. Such integrals appear frequently in probability theory.

Sample: A selected subset of a population, chosen by some process, usually with the objective of investigating particular properties of the parent population.

Sample size: The number of individuals to be included in an investigation. Usually chosen so that the study has a particular *power* of detecting an effect of a particular size. Software is available for calculating sample size for many types of study, for example, *SOLO*. See also **nomogram**.

Sample size formulae: Formulae for calculating the necessary sample size to achieve a given *power* of detecting an effect of some fixed magnitude. For example, the formula for determining the number of observations needed in each of two samples when using a *one-tailed z-test* to test for a difference in the means of two populations is:

$$n = \frac{2(z_\alpha - z_\beta)^2 \sigma^2}{(\mu_1 - \mu_2)^2}$$

where σ^2 is the known variance of each population, μ_1 and μ_2 the population means, z_α the *normal deviate* for the chosen significance level α, and z_β the normal deviate for β, where $1 - \beta$ is the required power. See also **SOLO**.

Sample survey: A study to estimate particular population characteristics using the information on the characteristics found from a sample of observations taken from the population. See also **opinion survey, random sample** and **quota sample**.

Sampling distribution: The *probability distribution* of a statistic. For example, the sampling distribution of the arithmetic mean of samples of size n, taken from a *normal distribution* with mean μ and standard deviation σ, is a normal distribution also with mean μ but with standard deviation $\sigma/\sqrt{n}$.

Sampling error: The difference between the sample result and the population characteristic being estimated. In practice, the sampling error can rarely be determined because the population characteristic is not usually known. With appropriate sampling procedures, however, it can be kept small, and the investigator can determine its probable limits of magnitude. See also **standard error**.

Sampling variation: The variation shown by different samples of the same size from the same population.

Sampling with and without replacement: Terms used to describe two possible methods of taking samples from a *finite population*. When each element is replaced before the next one is drawn, sampling is said to be 'with replacement'. When elements are not replaced, then the sampling is referred to as 'without replacement'. See also **bootstrap**, **jackknife** and **hypergeometric distribution**.

Sampling zeros: Zero frequencies that occur in the cells of *contingency tables* simply as a result of inadequate sample size. See also **structural zeros**.

Sandwich estimators: A term for estimators of covariances and variances, in the context of the *generalized estimating equation* approach to the analysis of *longitudinal studies* involving *categorical variables*. Such estimators are of the form

$$ABA$$

where the outside pieces of the 'sandwich' (the As) correspond to the value of the covariance which would have been obtained if the working correlations assumption were correct, and the centre terms (the B) depend on the true correlations of the responses.

SAS: An acronym for Statistical Analysis System, a large computer software system for data processing and data analysis. It contains extensive data management, file handling and graphics facilities, and can be used for most types of statistical analysis, including *regression analysis*, *log-linear models* and *principal components analysis*.

Saturated model: A model that contains all *main effects* and all possible *interactions* between factors. Since such a model contains the same number of parameters as observations, it results in a perfect fit for a data set.

Scalar: A single number, for example, 4, 10, 3.1, as opposed to a collection of numbers given in a vector or matrix.

Scaled deviance: A term used in *generalized linear models* for the *deviance* divided by the *scale factor*. Equals the deviance unless *overdispersion* is being modelled.

Scale factor: See **generalized linear models**.

Scales of measurement: A term used for the different levels of measurement used in medical investigations, these ranging from *categorical variables* through *ordinal variables* and *interval variables* to *ratio variables*. See also **clinimetrics** and **sensibility**.

Scan statistic: A statistic for evaluating whether an apparent *disease cluster* in time is due to chance. The statistic employs a 'moving window' of a particular length, and finds the maximum number of cases revealed through the window as it moves over the entire time period. Approximations for an upper bound to the probability of observing a certain size cluster under the null hypothesis of a *uniform distribution* are available. The statistic has been applied to test for possible clustering of lung cancer at a chemical works, rashes following injection of a varicella virus vaccine, and trisomic spontaneous abortions. See also **geographical analysis machine**.

Scatter: Synonym for **dispersion**.

Scatter diagram: A two-dimensional plot of a sample of bivariate observations. The diagram is an important aid in assessing what type of relationship links the two variables. See also **correlation coefficient** and **draughtsman's plot**. (See Fig. 58 opposite.)

Scattergram: Synonym for **scatter diagram**.

Scatterplot: Synonym for **scatter diagram**.

Sceptical priors: See **prior distributions**.

Scheffé's test: A *multiple comparison test* which protects against a large *per-experiment error rate*. In an *analysis of variance* of a *one way design*, for example, the method calculates the confidence interval for the difference between two means as

$$\bar{y}_{i.} - \bar{y}_{j.} \pm \sqrt{(g-1)F_{g-1,N-g}}\sqrt{MSE\left(\frac{1}{n_i}+\frac{1}{n_j}\right)}$$

where $\bar{y}_{i.}$ and $\bar{y}_{j.}$ are the observed means of groups i and j, g is the number of groups, MSE is the *error mean square* in the *analysis of variance table*, n_i and n_j are the number of observations in groups i and j, and $F_{g-1,N-g}$ is the F-value for some chosen significance level. The total sample size is represented by N.

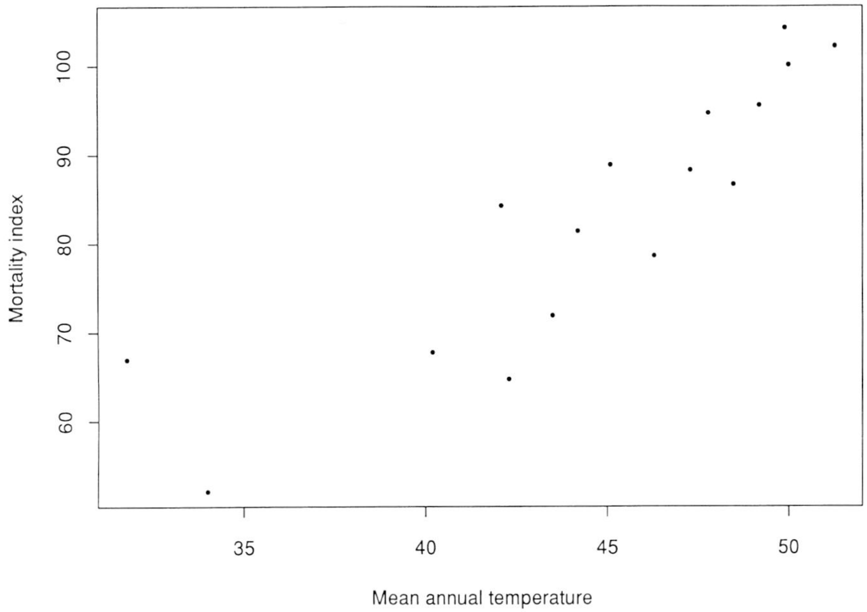

Fig 58 Scatter diagram for breast cancer mortality and region temperature.

Schoenfield residual: A diagnostic used in applications of *Cox's proportional hazards model*. This type of *residual* is not, in fact, a single value for each subject but a set of values, one for each explanatory variable included in the fitted model. Each such residual is the difference between the jth explanatory variable and a weighted average of the values of the explanatory variables over individuals in the *risk set* at the death time of the ith individual. The residuals have the properties that in large samples their *expected values* are zero and that they are uncorrelated with one another.

Schwarz's criterion: An index used as an aid in choosing between competing models. It is defined as

$$-2L_m + m \ln n$$

where n is the sample size, L_m is the maximized *log-likelihood* of the model and m is the number of parameters in the model. The index takes into account both the statistical goodness-of-fit and the number of parameters that have to be estimated to achieve this particular degree of fit, by imposing a penalty for increasing the number of parameters. Lower values of the index indicate the preferred model, that is, the one with the fewest parameters that still provides an adequate fit to the data. If $n \geq 8$ this criterion will tend to favour models with fewer parameters than those chosen by *Akaike's information criterion*. See also **parsimony principle** and **Occam's razor**.

Score residual: Synonym for **Schoenfield residual**.

Score test: A test for the hypothesis that a vector of parameters, $\boldsymbol{\theta}' = [\theta_1, \theta_2, \cdots, \theta_m]$, is the *null vector*. The test statistic is

$$s = \mathbf{s}'\mathbf{V}\mathbf{s}$$

where **s** is the vector with elements $\partial L / \partial \theta_i$ and L is the *log-likelihood*. **V** is the asymptotic *variance–covariance matrix* of the parameters. See also **Wald's test**.

Screened-to-eligible ratio: The number of subjects that have to be examined in a *clinical trial* to identify one protocol-eligible subject.

Screening studies: Studies in which *diagnostic tests* are applied to a symptomless population in order to diagnose disease at an early stage. Such studies are designed both to estimate disease *prevalence* and to identify for treatment patients who have particular diseases. The procedure is usually concerned with chronic illness and aims to detect disease not yet under medical care. Such studies need to be carefully designed and analyzed in order to avoid possible problems arising because of *lead time bias* and *length biased sampling*. Most suitable designs are based on *random allocation*. For example, in the *continuous screen design* subjects are randomized either to a group that are given periodic screening throughout the study, or to a group that do not get such screening but simply follow the usual medical care practices. One drawback of this type of design is that the cost involved in screening all the patients in the 'intervention' arm of the trial for the duration of the trial may be prohibitive; if this is so an alternative approach can be used, namely the *stop screen design*, in which screening is offered only for a limited time in the intervention group.

Scree plot: A plot of the ordered *eigenvalues* of a *correlation matrix*, used to indicate the appropriate number of factors in a *factor analysis*. The critical feature sought in the plot is an 'elbow', the number of factors then being taken as the number of eigenvalues up to this point. (See Fig. 59.)

SD: Abbreviation for **standard deviation**.

SE: Abbreviation for **standard error**.

Seasonally adjusted: A term applied to *time series* from which periodic oscillations with a period of one year have been removed.

Seasonal variation: Although strictly used to indicate the cycles in a *time series* that occur yearly, also often used to indicate other periodic movements.

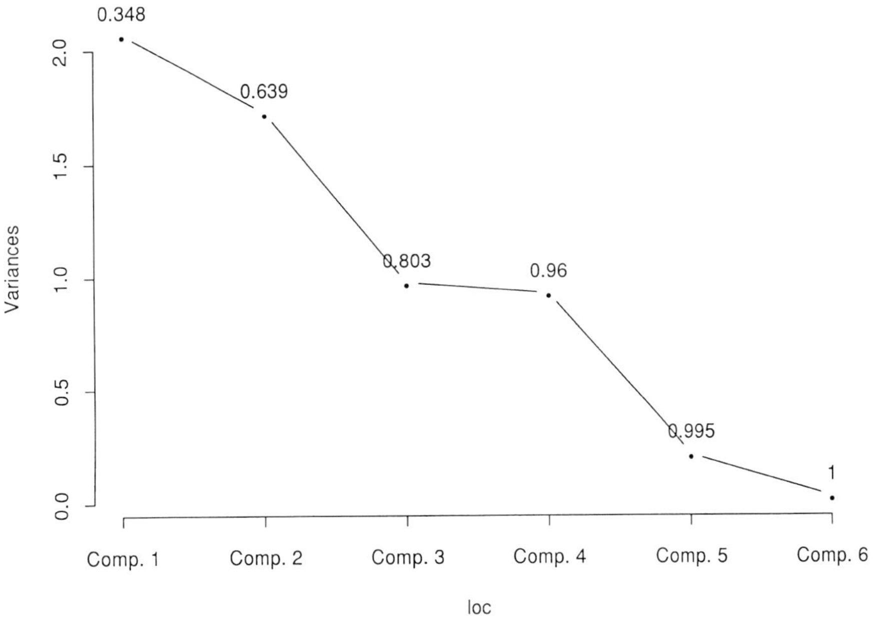

Fig 59 Scree plot showing an 'elbow' at eigenvalue three.

Secondary attack rate: The degree to which members of some collective or isolated unit, such as a household, litter or colony, become infected with a disease as a result of coming into contact with another member of the collective unit who became infected.

Secular trend: The underlying smooth movement of a *time series* over a fairly long period of time.

Selection bias: The bias that may be introduced into *clinical trials* and other types of medical investigations, whenever a treatment is chosen by the individual involved or is subject to constraints that go unobserved by the researcher. If there are unobserved factors influencing health outcomes and the type of treatment chosen, any direct links between treatment and outcome are confounded with unmeasured variables in the data. A classic example of this problem occurred in the Lanarkshire milk experiment of the 1920s. In this trial, 10 000 children were given free milk supplementation and a similar number received no supplementation. The groups were formed by *random allocation*. Unfortunately however, well-intentioned teachers decided that the poorest children should be given priority for free milk rather than sticking strictly to the original groups. The consequence was that the effects of milk supplementation were indistinguishable from the effects of poverty.

Selection methods in regression: A series of methods for selecting 'good' (although not necessarily the best) subsets of explanatory variables when using *regression analysis*. The three most commonly used of these methods are *forward selection, backward elimination*, and a combination of both of these known as *stepwise regression*. The criterion used for assessing whether or not a variable should be added to an existing model in forward selection or removed from an existing model in backward elimination is, essentially, the change in the *residual sum of squares* produced by the inclusion or exclusion of the variable. Specifically, in forward selection, an 'F-statistic' known as the *F-to-enter*, is calculated as

$$F = \frac{RSS_m - RSS_{m+1}}{RSS_{m+1}/(n-m-2)}$$

and compared with a preset term; calculated Fs greater than the preset value lead to the variable under consideration being added to the model. (RSS_m and RSS_{m+1} are the residual sums of squares when models with m and $m+1$ explanatory variables have been fitted). In backward selection, a calculated F less than a corresponding *F-to-remove* leads to a variable being removed from the current model. In the stepwise procedure, variables are entered as with forward selection, but after each addition of a new variable, those variables currently in the model are considered for removal by the backward elimination process. In this way it is possible that variables included at some earlier stage might later be removed, because the presence of new variables has made their contribution to the regression model no longer important. It should be stressed that none of these automatic procedures for selecting variables is foolproof and they must be used with care. See also **all subsets regression**.

Self-pairing: See **paired samples**.

Semantic differential scale: A scale for eliciting ratings of a particular concept on a series of dimensions. For example,

My treatment is

Painful – Painless
Helpful – Not helpful

See also **visual analogue scale**.

Semi-interquartile range: Half the difference between the upper and lower *quartiles*.

Sensibility: A term used in the context of constructing scales for measuring clinical phenomena that relates to how appropriate or 'sensible' the proposed scale is likely to be. The qualitative judgements used in the evaluation of the sensibility of a scale include:

- the purpose and framework for which the scale is intended: what are its clinical function, clinical justification and clinical applicability?
- is the scale comprehensible, simple, thorough and clear in its direction for usage?
- is the scale aimed at the right thing? Is it put together in the right way?
- have important variables been omitted from or unsuitable variables been included in the scale? Have suitable score ranges and weights been used for the component variables of the scale? How good is the quality of the basic data used in assigning scores?
- how much time and effort is required to obtain and organize the data needed for the scale?

Sensitivity: An index of the performance of a *diagnostic test*, calculated as the percentage of individuals with a disease who are correctly classified as having the disease, i.e., the *conditional probability* of having a positive test result, given having the disease. A test is sensitive to the disease if it is positive for most individuals having the disease. See also **specificity** and **Bayes' theorem**.

Sensitivity analysis: See **uncertainty analysis**.

Sequential analysis: A procedure in which a statistical test of significance is conducted repeatedly over time as the data are collected. After each observation, the cumulative data are analysed and one of the following three decisions taken:

- stop the data collection, reject the *null hypothesis* and claim statistical significance;
- stop the data collection, do not reject the null hypothesis and state that the results are not statistically significant;
- continue the data collection, since as yet the cumulated data are inadequate to draw a conclusion.

In some cases, *open sequential designs*, no provision is made to terminate the trial with the conclusion that there is no difference between the treatments, in others, *closed sequential designs*, such a conclusion can be reached. In *group sequential designs*, *interim analyses* are undertaken after each accumulation of a particular number of subjects into the two groups. Suitable values for the number of subjects can be found from the overall significance level, the expected treatment difference and the required *power*.

Sequential sums of squares: A term encountered primarily in *regression analysis* for the contributions of variables as they are added to the model in a particular sequence. Essentially, the difference in the *residual sum of squares* before and after adding a variable.

Serial correlation: Synonym for **autocorrelation**.

Serial dilution assay: A standard microbiological method for estimating the density (average number of organisms per unit volume) in a solution, under the assumptions:

- that the organisms are randomly distributed throughout the solution;
- that each sample from the solution, when incubated in the culture medium, is certain to exhibit fertility whenever the sample contains one or more organisms.

Maximum likelihood estimation is used to provide an estimate of the solution average organisms per unit volume, which is usually known as the *most probable number*.

Serial interval: The period from the observation of symptoms in one case to the observation of symptoms in a second case directly infected from the first.

Serial measurements: Observations on the same subject collected over time. See also **longitudinal data**.

Serologic data: Data produced in studies where the presence of antibodies in individuals is investigated using a serological test. For example, the proportion of individuals in different age groups who are seropositive may be recorded.

Sets technique: A procedure for the detection of low-level epidemics of rare diseases such as birth defects and cancer. Analysis of the time intervals between each of the last n cases is carried out each time a new case is diagnosed. An alarm is signalled if each of the n intervals is shorter than a given reference value. See also **cusum**.

Shaded distance matrix: A rough but simple way of graphically displaying a solution obtained from a *cluster analysis* of a set of observations, so that the effectiveness of the solution can be assessed. The individuals are rearranged so that those in the same cluster are adjacent to one another in the distance matrix. Distances within a cluster will be small for tight and well separated clusters, while the distances between individuals in different clusters will be large. Coding increasing distance by decreasing gray levels should result in a series of dark triangles under each tight well separated cluster, while clusters that are simply artifacts of the clustering procedure will not exhibit such behaviour. (See Fig. 60 opposite.)

Shannon's information measure: A measure of the average information in an event with probability P, given by

$$(-\log P)$$

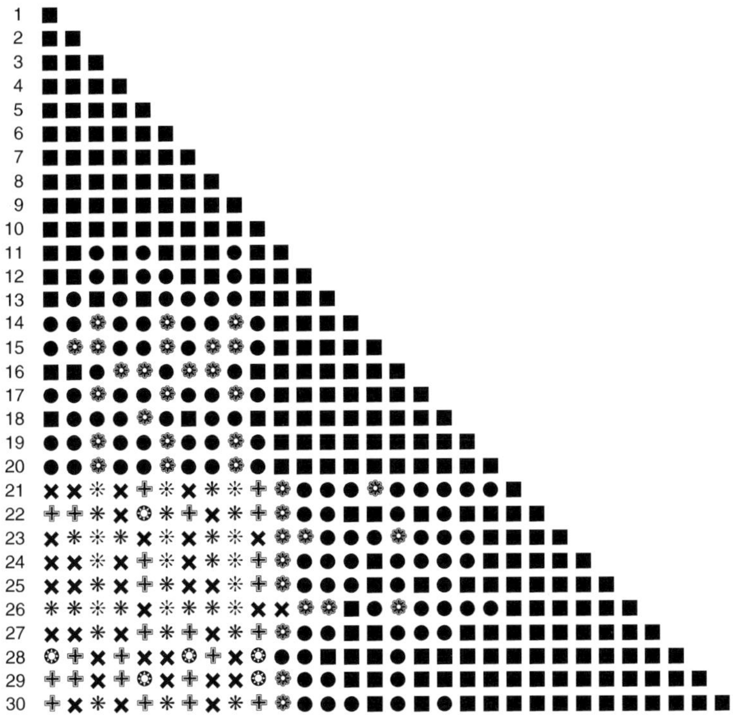

Fig 60 An example of a shaded distance matrix.

The measure is intuitively reasonable, in the sense that the more unlikely the event, the more information is provided by the knowledge that the event has occurred. The presence of a logarithm ensures that the information is additive. The logarithmic base is arbitrary and determines the unit of information. Usually base 2 is used so that information is measured in *bits*. See also **information theory** and index of **entropy**.

Shapiro–Wilk W tests: Tests that a set of *random variables* arise from a specified *probability distribution*. Most commonly used to test for departures from the *normal distribution* and the *exponential distribution*. For the latter, the *test statistic* is

$$W = \frac{n}{n-1} \frac{(\bar{x} - x_{(1)})^2}{\sum_{i=1}^{n} (x_{(i)} - \bar{x})^2}$$

where $x_{(1)} \leq x_{(2)} \cdots \leq x_{(n)}$ are the ordered sample values and $\bar{x}$ is their mean. Critical values of W based on *simulation* studies are available in many statistical tables.

Shelf-life: The time interval that a drug product is expected to remain within the approved specifications after manufacture.

Shepard diagram: A type of plot used in *multidimensional scaling*, in which observed *dissimilarity coefficients* are plotted against the distances derived from the scaling solution. By joining together consecutive points in the diagram, insight can be gained into the transformation needed to convert the observed dissimilarities into distances.

Sheppard's corrections: Adjustments to improve the estimates of population *moments* obtained from the corresponding sample moments calculated from grouped data. The correction is used to overcome the error introduced by assuming that all the values in a class in the grouped data take the same value as the class mid-point.

Shrinkage: The phenomenon that generally occurs when an equation derived from, say, a *multiple regression*, is applied to a new data set, in which the model predicts much less well than in the original sample. In particular, the value of the *multiple correlation coefficient* becomes less, i.e., it 'shrinks'.

Sickness absence: Absence from work attributed to medical incapacity.

Sigmoid: A description of a curve having an elongated 'S'-shape.

Signed rank test: See **Wilcoxon's signed rank test**.

Significance level: The level of probability at which it is agreed that the *null hypothesis* will be rejected. Conventionally set at 0.05.

Significance test: A statistical procedure that, when applied to a set of observations, results in a *P-value* relative to some hypothesis. Examples include *Student's t-test*, *z-test* and *Wilcoxon's signed rank test*.

Sign test: A test of the *null hypothesis* that positive and negative values amongst a series of observations are equally likely. The observations are often differences between a response variable observed under two conditions on a set of subjects.

Similarity coefficient: Coefficients, ranging usually from zero to unity used to measure the similarity of the variable values of two observations from a set of *multivariate data*. Most commonly used on *binary variables*. Example of such coefficients are the *matching coefficient* and *Jaccard's coefficient*.

Similarity matrix: A *symmetric matrix* in which values on the main diagonal are unity, and off-diagonal elements are the values of some *similarity coefficient* for the corresponding pair of individuals.

Simple structure: See **factor analysis**.

Simplex algorithm: A procedure for maximizing or minimizing a function of several variables. The basic idea behind the algorithm is to compare the values of the function being minimized at the vertices of a simplex in the parameter space, and to move this simplex gradually towards the minimum during the iterative process by a combination of reflection, contraction and expansion.

Simpson's paradox: The observation that a measure of association between two variables (for example, type of treatment and outcome) may be identical within the levels of a third variable (for example, sex), but can take on an entirely different value when the third variable is disregarded, and the association measure calculated from the pooled data. Such a situation can only occur if the third variable is associated with both of the other two variables. As an example, consider the following pair of *two-by-two contingency tables* giving information about amount of prenatal care and survival in two clinics:

Clinic A

		Infant's survival		
		Died	Survived	Total
	Less	3	176	179
Amount of care	More	4	293	279
	Total	7	469	476

Clinic B

		Infant's survival		
		Died	Survived	Total
	Less	17	197	214
Amount of care	More	2	23	25
	Total	19	220	239

In both clinics, A and B, the *chi-squared statistic* for assessing the hypothesis of independence of survival and amount of care leads to acceptance of the hypothesis. (In both cases the statistic is almost zero.) If, however the data are collapsed over clinics the resulting chi-squared statistic takes the value 5.26, and the conclusion would now be that amount of care and survival are related. See also **collapsing categories** and **log-linear models**.

Simulated annealing: Synonym for **annealing algorithm**.

Simulation: The artificial generation of random processes (usually by means of *pseudorandom numbers* and/or computers) to imitate the behaviour of particular statistical models. See also **Monte Carlo methods**.

Simultaneous confidence interval: A *confidence interval* (perhaps more correctly a region) for several parameters being estimated simultaneously.

Single-blind: See **blinding**.

Single-case study: Synonym for **N of 1 clinical trial**.

Single linkage clustering: A method of *cluster analysis* in which the distance between two clusters is defined as the least distance between a pair of individuals, one member of the pair being in each group.

Single-masked: Synonym for **single blind**.

Single sample t**-test**: See **Student's** t**-tests**.

Singly censored data: *Censored observations* that occur in *clinical trials* where all the patients enter the study at the same time point, and where the study is terminated after a fixed time period. See also **progressively censored data**.

Singular matrix: A *square matrix* whose *determinant* is equal to zero; a matrix whose inverse is not defined.

Singular value decomposition: The decomposition of an $r \times c$ matrix, $\mathbf{A}$ into the form

$$\mathbf{A} = \mathbf{USV}'$$

where $\mathbf{U}$ and $\mathbf{V}'$ are *orthogonal matrices* and $\mathbf{S}$ is a *diagonal matrix*. The basis of several techniques of *multivariate analysis* including *correspondence analysis*.

Sister dependence: The dependence of the times from the division of a 'mother' cell to the division of each of the pair of 'sister' cells created by the mother cell division.

Skewness: The lack of symmetry in a *probability distribution*. Usually quantified by the index, s, given by

$$s = \frac{\mu_3}{\mu_2^{3/2}}$$

where μ_2 and μ_3 are the second and third *moments* about the mean. The index takes the value zero for a *symmetrical distribution*. A distribution is said to have *positive skewness* when it has a long thin tail at the right, and to have *negative skewness* when it has a long thin tail to the left.

Skew-symmetric matrix: A matrix in which the elements a_{ij} satisfy

$$a_{ii} = 0; \quad a_{ij} = -a_{ji}, \; i \neq j$$

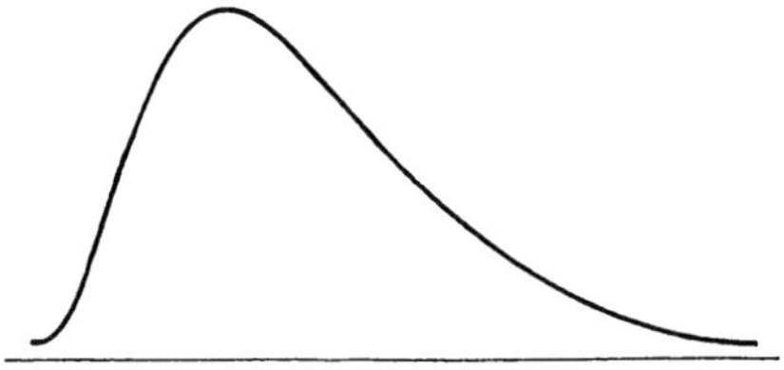

Distribution with positive skewness.

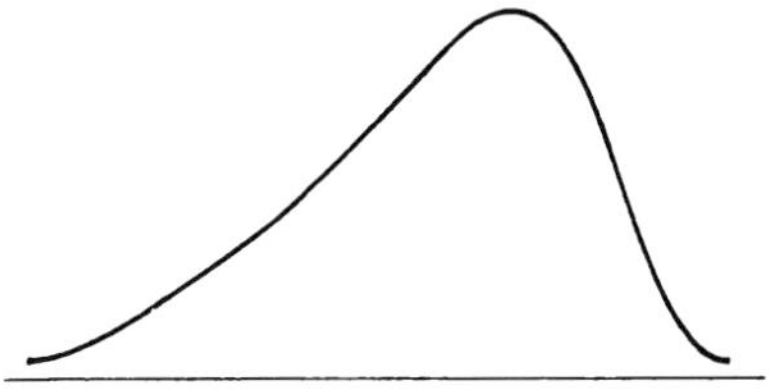

Distribution with negative skewness.

Fig 61 Positive and negative skewness.

An example of such a matrix is **A** given by

$$\mathbf{A} = \begin{pmatrix} 0 & 1 & -3 \\ -1 & 0 & 2 \\ 3 & -2 & 0 \end{pmatrix}$$

Sliding square plot: A graphical display of *paired samples* data. A scatterplot of the n pairs of observations (x_i, y_i) forms the basis of the plot, and this is enhanced by three *box-and-whisker plots*, one for the first observation in each pair (i.e., the control subject or the measurement taken on the first occasion), one for the remaining observation, and one for the differences between the pairs, i.e., $x_i - y_i$. (See Fig. 62 overleaf.)

Slope ratio assay: A general class of biological assay, where the *dose–response* lines for the standard test stimuli are not in the form of two parallel regression lines, but of two different lines with different slopes intersecting the ordinate at a point corresponding to zero doses of the stimuli. The relative potency of these stimuli is obtained by taking the ratio of the estimated slopes of the two lines.

Slutzky–Yule effect: The oscillatory series often produced when a *moving average* is applied to a *time series* consisting of random observations.

Small expected frequencies: A term that is found in discussions of the analysis of *contingency tables*. It arises because the derivation of the *chi-squared*

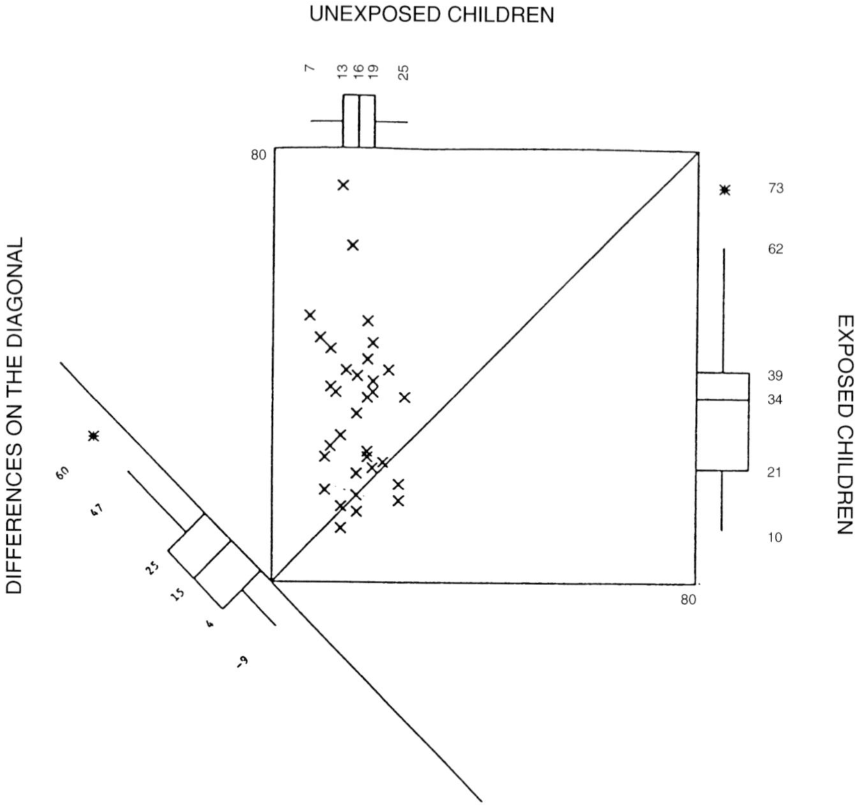

Fig 62 An example of a sliding square plot for blood lead levels of matched pairs of children.

distribution, as an approximation for the distribution of the *chi-squared statistic* when the hypothesis of independence is true, is made under the assumption that the *expected frequencies* are not too small. Typically, this rather vague phrase has been interpreted as meaning that a satisfactory approximation is achieved only when expected frequencies are five or more. Despite the widespread acceptance of this 'rule', it is nowadays thought to be largely irrelevant, since there is a great deal of evidence that the usual chi-squared statistic can be used safely when expected frequencies are far smaller. See also **STATXACT**.

Smear-and-sweep: A method of adjusting death rates for the effects of confounding variables. The procedure is iterative, each iteration consisting of two steps. The first entails 'smearing' the data into a two-way classification based on two of the confounding variables, and the second consisists of 'sweeping' the resulting cells into categories according to their ordering on the death rate of interest.

Smoothing: The removal of minor fluctuations from a series of observations, usually by applying some form of *regression analysis*, particularly *locally weighted regression*.

SMR: Acronym for **standardized mortality rate**.

Snedecor's F-distribution: Synonym for **F-distribution**.

Snowball sampling: A method of sampling that uses sample members to provide names of other potential sample members. For example, in sampling heroin addicts, an addict may be asked for the names of other addicts that he or she knows. Little is known about the statistical properties of such samples.

Snowflakes: A graphical technique for displaying *multivariate data*. For q variables, a snowflake is constructed by plotting the magnitude of each variable along equiangular rays originating from the same point. Each observation corresponds to a particular shaped snowflake and these are often displayed side-by-side for quick visual inspection. See also **Andrews' plots, Chernoff's faces** and **glyphs**.

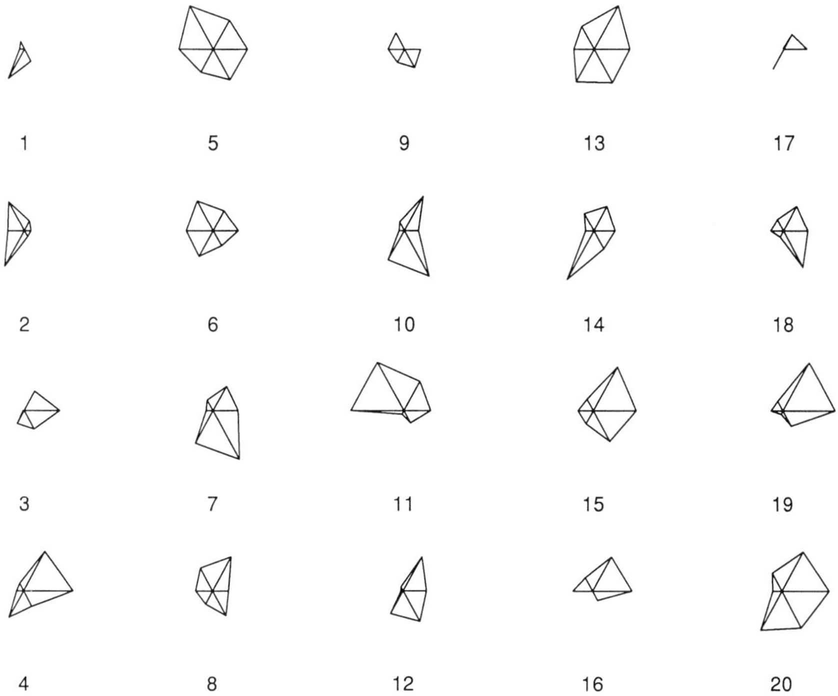

Fig 63 A set of snowflakes for twenty six-dimensional multivariate observations.

Sojourn time: Most often used for the interval during which a particular condition is potentially detectable but not yet diagnosed, but also occurs in the context of *Markov chains* as the number of times state k, say, is visited in the first n transitions.

SOLO: A computer package for calculating sample sizes to achieve a particular *power* for a variety of different research designs.

Somer's d: A measure of association for a *contingency table* with ordered row and column categories, that is suitable for the asymmetric case in which one variable is considered the response and one explanatory. See also **Kendall's tau statistics**.

Sources of data: Usually refers to reports and government publications giving, for example, statistics on cancer registrations, number of abortions carried out in particular time periods, or number of deaths from AIDS. Examples of such reports are those provided by the World Health Organization, such as the *World Health Statistics Annual*, which details the seasonal distribution of new cases for about forty different infectious diseases, and the *World Health Quarterly*, which includes statistics on *mortality* and *morbidity*.

Space–time clustering: An approach to the analysis of epidemics that takes account of three components:

- the time distribution of cases;
- the space distribution;
- a measure of the space–time interaction.

The analysis uses the simultaneous measurement and classification of time and distance intervals between all possible pairs of cases.

Spatial data: A collection of measurements or observations on one or more variables, taken at specified locations, and for which the spatial organization of the data is of primary interest.

Spatial median: An extension of the concept of a median to *bivariate data*. Defined as the value of θ that minimizes the measure of scatter, $T(\theta)$, given by

$$T(\theta) = \sum ||\boldsymbol{x}_i - \theta||$$

where $||\quad||$ is the *Euclidean distance* and $\mathbf{x}_1, \mathbf{x}_2, \cdots, \mathbf{x}_n$ are n bivariate observations. See also **bivariate Oja median**.

Spatial randomness: See **complete spatial randomness**.

Spearman–Karber estimator: An estimator of the *median effective dose* in bioassays having a *binary variable* as a response.

Spearman's rho: A *rank correlation coefficient*. If the ranked values of the two variables for a set of n individuals are a_i and b_i, with $d_i = a_i - b_i$, then the coefficient is defined explicitly as

$$\rho = 1 - \frac{6\sum_{i=1}^{n} d_i^2}{n^3 - n}$$

In essence ρ is simply *Pearson's product moment correlation coefficient* between the rankings a and b. See also **Kendall's tau statistics**.

Specificity: An index of the performance of a *diagnostic test*, calculated as the percentage of individuals without the disease who are classified as not having the disease, i.e., the *conditional probability* of a negative test result given that the disease is absent. A test is specific if it is positive for only a small percentage of those without the disease. See also **sensitivity** and **Bayes' theorem**.

Specific variates: See **factor analysis**.

Spectral analysis: A procedure for the analysis of the frequencies and periodicities in *time series* data. The time series is effectively decomposed into an infinite number of periodic components, each of infinitesimal amplitude, so the purpose of the analysis is to estimate the contributions of components in certain ranges of frequency. Such an analysis may show that contributions to the fluctuations in the time series come from a continuous range of frequencies, and the pattern of spectral densities may suggest a particular model for the series. Alternatively, the analysis may suggest one or two dominant frequencies. See also **harmonic analysis** and **periodogram**.

Sphericity: See **Mauchly test**.

Spline function: A smoothly joined piecewise polynomial of degree n. For example, if $t_1, t_2, \cdots, t_n$ are a set of n values in the interval (a,b), such that $a < t_1 \leq t_2 \cdots \leq t_n \leq b$, then a *cubic spline* is a function g such that on each of the intervals $(a, t_1), (t_1, t_2), \cdots, (t_n, b)$, g is a cubic polynomial, and secondly the polynomial pieces fit together at the points t_i in such a way that g itself and its first and second derivatives are continuous at each t_i and hence on the whole of (a,b). The points t_i are called *knots*. Such curves are widely used for *interpolation* and in some forms of *regression analysis*.

Split-half method: A procedure used primarily in psychology to estimate the reliability of a test. Two scores are obtained from the same test, either from alternative items, the so-called odd-even technique, or from parallel sections of items. The correlation of these scores, or some transformation of them, gives the required reliability. See also **Cronbach's alpha**.

Split-plot design: A term originating in agricultural field experiments, where the division of a testing area or 'plot' into a number of parts permitted the inclusion of an extra factor into the study. In medicine, similar designs occur when the same patient or subject is observed at each level of a factor, or at all combinations of levels of a number of factors. See also **longitudinal data**.

S-PLUS: A high level programming language with extensive graphical and statistical features that can be used to undertake both standard and non-standard analyses relatively simply.

Spread: Synonym for **dispersion**.

Spreadsheet: In computer technology, a two-way table, with entries which may be numbers or text. Facilities include operations on rows or columns. Entries may also give references to other entries, making possible more complex operations.

SPSS: A statistical software package, an acronym for Statistical Package for the Social Sciences. A comprehensive range of statistical procedures is available and, in addition, extensive facilities for file manipulation and recoding or transforming data.

Spurious correlation: A term usually reserved for the introduction of correlation due to computing rates using the same denominator. Specifically, if two variables X and Y are not related, then the two ratios X/Z and Y/Z will be related.

Spurious precision: The tendency to report results to too many significant figures, largely due to copying figures directly from computer output without applying some sensible *rounding*.

Square contingency table: A *contingency table* with the same number of rows as columns.

Square matrix: A matrix with the same number of rows as columns. *Variance–covariance matrices* and *correlation matrices* are statistical examples.

Square root transformation: A transformation of the form $y = \sqrt{x}$, often used to make *random variables* suspected to have a *Poisson distribution* more suitable for techniques such as *analysis of variance*, by making their variances independent of their means. See also **variance stabilizing transformations**.

Stability analysis: A term usually applied to investigations carried out by pharmaceutical companies to determine the *shelf-life* of their drug products. The procedure generally involves testing various batches of the product at several storage time points.

Staircase method: Synonym for **up-and-down method**.

Standard curve: The curve which relates the responses in an assay given by a range of standard solutions to their known concentrations. It permits the analytic concentration of an unknown solution to be inferred from its assay response by *interpolation*.

Standard design: Synonym for **Fibonacci dose escalation scheme**.

Standard deviation (SD): The most commonly used measure of the spread of a set of observations. Equal to the square root of the *variance*.

Standard error (SE): The *standard deviation* of the *sampling distribution* of a statistic. For example, the standard error of the sample mean of n observations is $\sigma/\sqrt{n}$, where σ^2 is the variance of the original observations.

Standardization: A term used in a variety of ways in medical research. The most common usage is in the context of transforming a variable by dividing by its *standard deviation* to give a new variable with standard deviation unity. Also often used for the process of producing an index of mortality, which is adjusted for the age distribution in a particular group being examined. See also **standardized mortality rate, indirect standardization** and **direct standardization**.

Standardized mortality rate (SMR): The number of deaths, either total or cause-specific, in a given population, expressed as a percentage of the deaths that would have been expected if the age and sex-specific rates in a 'standard' population had applied.

Standardized regression coefficient: See **beta coefficient**.

Standardized residual: See **residual**.

Standard normal distribution: A *normal distribution* with zero mean and unit variance.

Standard normal variable: A *random* variable having a *standard normal distribution.*

Standard scores: Variable values transformed to zero mean and unit variance.

Stationary series: A *time series*, $\{x_t\}$, with mean and variance that are independent of t.

Statistic: A numerical characteristic of a sample. For example, the sample mean and sample variance. See also **parameter**.

Statistical expert system: A computer program that leads a user through a valid statistical analysis, choosing suitable tools by examining the data and interrogating the user, and explaining its actions, decisions, and conclusions on request.

Statistical software: A set of computer programs implementing commonly used statistical methods. See also **BMDP, GLIM, GENSTAT, MINITAB, SAS, S-PLUS, SPSS** and **EGRET**.

Statistical surveillance: The continual observation of a *time series* with the goal of detecting an important change in the underlying process as soon as possible after it has occurred. An example of where such a procedure is of considerable importance is in monitoring foetal heart rate during labour.

STATXACT: A specialised statistical package for analysing data from *contingency tables* that provides exact *P-values*, which, in the case of sparse tables, may differ considerable from the values given by *asymptotic statistics* such as the *chi-squared statistic*.

```
14 : 2
14 : 555
14 : 67777
14 : 889
15 : 000000111111
15 : 22222222222233333333333333333
15 : 44444444444555555555555555555555
15 : 6666666666666666666677777777777777777777
15 : 888888888888888888888888888888899999999999999999
16 : 00000000000000000000011111111111111111111
16 : 222222222222222222333333333333333333333333333333
16 : 44444444444444444555555555555555555
16 : 666666666667777777
16 : 88888899999999
17 : 00000000000111
17 : 333
17 : 4
17 : 67
17 : 88
```

Fig 64 A stem-and-leaf display of the heights (cm) of 351 elderly women.

Steepest descent: A procedure for finding the maximum or minimum value of a function of several variables, by searching in the direction of the negative gradient of the function with respect to the parameters. See also **simplex method** and **Newton–Raphson method**.

Stem-and-leaf plot: A method of displaying data in which each observation is split into two parts, labelled the 'stem' and the 'leaf', for example, tens and units. The stems are arranged in a column, and leaves are attached to the relevant stem. The resulting display gives the shape information usually provided by a *histogram*, whilst retaining the original observation values. See also **back-to-back stem-and-leaf plot**.

Stepwise regression: See **selection methods in regression**.

Stillbirth rate: The number of stillbirths divided by the number of live and stillbirths in the same time period. Usually expressed per 1000 total births per year. The following table gives the rates for England, Wales, Scotland and Northern Ireland for both 1971 and 1992.

	1971	**1992**
England	12.4	4.2
Wales	14.2	4.1
Scotland	13.1	5.4
Northern Ireland	14.3	4.7

Stochastic process: A series of *random variables*, $\{x_t\}$, where t assumes values in a certain range T. In most cases x_t is an observation at time t and T is a time range.

Stopping rules: Procedures that allow *interim analyses* in *clinical trials* at predefined times, whilst preserving the *type I error* at some pre-specified level. See also **sequential analysis**.

Stop screen design: See **screening studies**.

Strata: See **stratification**.

Stratification: The division of a population into parts known as *strata*, particularly for the purpose of drawing a sample.

Stratified logrank test: A method for comparing the survival experience of two groups of subjects given different treatments, when the groups are stratified by age or some other prognostic variable.

Stratified randomization: A procedure designed to allocate patients to treatments in clinical trials to achieve approximate balance of important characteristics, without sacrificing the advantages of *random allocation*. See also **minimization**.

Stratified random sampling: *Random sampling* from each *strata* of a population after *stratification*.

Stress: A term used for a particular measure of *goodness-of-fit* in *multidimensional scaling*.

Stroke index: A global measure of disease activity in rheumatoid arthritis. The index is based on two objective laboratory measurements, one subjective and two semi-objective clinical measurements, chosen from 13 possibilities by using clinical judgement.

Structural equation modelling: A procedure that combines aspects of *multiple regression* and *factor analysis*, to investigate relationships between *latent variables*. See also **LISREL** and **EQS**.

Structural zeros: Zero frequencies occurring in the cells of contingency tables which arise because it is theoretically impossible for an observation to fall in the cell. For example, if male and female students are asked about health problems that cause them concern, then the cell corresponding to, say, menstrual problems for men will have a zero entry. See also **sampling zeros**.

Stuart–Maxwell test: A test of *marginal homogeneity* in a *square contingency table*. The *test statistic* is given by

$$X^2 = \mathbf{d}'\mathbf{V}^{-1}\mathbf{d}$$

where $\mathbf{d}$ is a column vector of any $r-1$ differences of corresponding row and column marginal totals, with r being the number of rows and columns in the table. The $(r-1) \times (r-1)$ matrix $\mathbf{V}$ contains variances and covariances of these differences, i.e.,

$$v_{ii} = n_{i.} + n_{.j} - 2n_{ij}$$
$$v_{ij} = -(n_{ij} + n_{ji})$$

where n_{ij} are the observed frequencies in the table and $n_{i.}$ and $n_{.j}$ are marginal totals. If the hypothesis of marginal homogeneity is true, then X^2 has a *chi-squared distribution* with $r-1$ degrees of freedom.

Studentization: The removal of a *nuisance parameter* by constructing a statistic whose *sampling distribution* does not depend on that parameter.

Studentized range statistic: A statistic that occurs most often in *multiple comparison tests*. It is defined as

$$q = \frac{\bar{x}_{\text{largest}} - \bar{x}_{\text{smallest}}}{\sqrt{\text{MSE}/n}}$$

where $\bar{x}_{\text{largest}}$ and $\bar{x}_{\text{smallest}}$ are the largest and smallest means amongst the means of k groups, and MSE is the *error mean square* from an *analysis of variance* of the groups.

Studentized residual: See **residual.**

Student's t-distribution: The *probability distribution* of the ratio of a *standard normal variable* to the square root of a variable with a *chi-squared distribution.* In particular the distribution of the variable

$$t = \frac{\bar{x} - \mu}{s/\sqrt{n}}$$

where $\bar{x}$ is the arithmetic mean of n observations from a *normal distribution* with mean μ, and s is the sample standard deviation. The shape of the distribution varies with n, and as n gets larger the shape of the t-distribution approaches that of the *standard normal distribution.*

Student's t-tests: Significance tests for assessing hypotheses about population means. One version is used in situations where it is required to test whether the mean of a population takes a particular value. This is generally known as a *single sample t-test*. Another version is designed to test the equality of the means of two populations. When independent samples are available from each population, the procedure is often known as the *independent samples t-test*, and the *test statistic* is

$$t = \frac{\bar{x}_1 - \bar{x}_2}{s\sqrt{\frac{1}{n_1} + \frac{1}{n_2}}}$$

where $\bar{x}_1$ and $\bar{x}_2$ are the means of samples of size n_1 and n_2 taken from each population, and s^2 is an estimate of the assumed common variance, given by

$$s^2 = \frac{(n_1 - 1)s_1^2 + (n_2 - 1)s_2^2}{n_1 + n_2 - 2}$$

If the *null hypothesis* of the equality of the two population means is true, t has a *Student's t-distribution* with $n_1 + n_2 - 2$ degrees of freedom, allowing *P-values* to be calculated. The test assumes that each population has a *normal distribution*, but is known to be relatively insensitive to departures from this assumption. See also **matched pairs t-test**.

Sturdy statistics: Synonym for **robust statistics**.

Subgroup analysis: The analysis of particular subgroups of patients in a *clinical trial* to assess possible treatment–subgroup interactions. An investigator may, for example, want to understand whether a drug affects older patients differently from those who are younger. Analysing many subgroupings for treatment effects can greatly increase overall *type I error* rates. See also **fishing expedition** and **data dredging**.

Subjective endpoints: Endpoints in *clinical trials* that can only be measured by subjective clinical rating scales.

Subjective probability: Synonym for **personal probability**.

Sufficient statistic: A statistic that, in a certain sense, summarizes all the information contained in a sample of observations about a particular parameter.

Sullivan's index: An index in which morbidity data and information from *life tables* is combined to produce an estimate of illness-free life expectancy.

Sunflower plot: A modification of the usual *scatter diagram*, designed to reduce the problem of overlap caused by multiple points at one position (particularly if the data have been rounded to integers). The scatterplot is first partitioned with a grid and the number of points in each cell of the grid is counted. If there is only a single point in a cell, a dot is plotted at the centre of the cell. If there is more than one observation in a cell, a 'sunflower' icon is drawn on which the number of 'petals' is equal to the number of points falling in that cell.

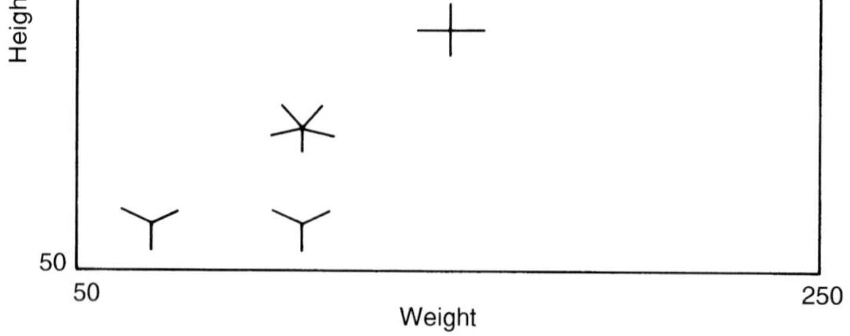

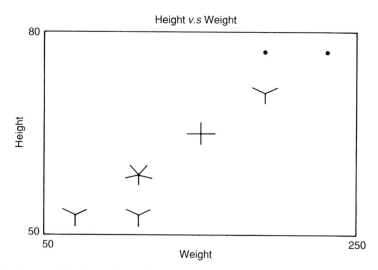

Fig 65 An example of a sunflower plot.

Supernormality: A term sometimes used in the context of *normal probability plots* of *residuals* from, for example, a *regression analysis*. Because such residuals are *linear functions* of *random variables*, they will tend to be more normal than the underlying error distribution, if this is not normal. Thus, a straight plot does not necessarily mean that the error distribution is normal. Consequently, the main use of probability plots of this kind should be for the detection of unduly influential or outlying observations.

Supervised pattern recognition: See **pattern recognition**.

Support: A term often used for the *likelihood*, to stress its role as a measure of the evidence produced by a set of observations for a particular value(s) of the parameter(s) of a model.

Suppressor variables: A variable in a *regression analysis* that is not correlated with the dependent variable, but that is still useful for increasing the size of the *multiple correlation coefficient* by virtue of its correlations with other explanatory variables. The variable 'suppresses' variance that is irrelevant to prediction of the dependent variable.

Surface models: A term used for those models for *screening studies* that consider only those events that can be directly observed, such as disease *incidence*, *prevalence* and *mortality*. See also **deep models**.

Surrogate endpoint: A term often encountered in discussions of *clinical trials* to refer to an outcome measure that an investigator considers is highly correlated with an endpoint of interest, but that can be measured at lower expense or at an earlier time. In some cases, ethical issues may suggest the use of a surrogate. Examples include measurement of blood pressure as a surrogate for cardiovascular mortality, lipid levels as a surrogate for arteriosclerosis, and, in cancer studies, time to relapse as a surrogate for total survival time. Considerable controversy in interpretation can be generated when doubts arise about the correlation of the surrogate endpoint with the endpoint of interest, or over whether or not the surrogate endpoint should be considered as an endpoint of primary interest in its own right.

Surrogate observation: An observed variable that relates in some way to the variable of primary importance, which cannot itself be conveniently observed directly. See also **latent variable**.

Survey: An investigation that collects planned information from individuals about their history, habits, knowledge, attitudes or behaviour.

Survival curve: See **survival function**.

Survival function: The probability that the *survival time* of an individual is longer than some particular value. A plot of this probability against time is called a *survival curve* and is a useful component in the analysis of such data. See also **product limit estimator** and **hazard function**.

Survival time: Observations of the time until the occurrence of a particular event, for example, recovery, improvement or death.

Survivor function: Synonym for **survival function**.

Suspended rootogram: Synonym for **hanging rootogram**.

Symmetrical distribution: A *probability distribution* or *frequency distribution* that is symmetrical about some central value.

Symmetric matrix: A *square matrix* that is symmetrical about its leading diagonal, i.e., a matrix with elements a_{ij} such that $a_{ij} = a_{ji}$. In statistics, *correlation matrices* and *variance–covariance matrices* are of this form.

Symmetry in square contingency tables: See **Bowker's test for symmetry**.

Symptom checklist: A brief multidimensional self-report inventory designed to screen for a broad range of psychological problems and symtoms of psychopathology. It can be useful in the initial evaluation of patients as an objective method of screening for psychological problems and to measure patient progress during treatment. See also **general health questionnaire**.

Synergism: A term used when the joint effect of two treatments is greater than the sum of their effects when administered separately (*positive synergism*), or when the sum of their effects is less than when administered separately (*negative synergism or antagonism*).

Synthetic risk maps: Plots of the principal component scores derived from a *principal components analysis* of the correlations among cancer mortality rates at different body sites.

SYSTAT: A comprehensive statistical software package with particularly good graphical facilities.

Systematic allocation: Procedures for allocating treatments to patients in a *clinical trial*, that attempt to emulate *random allocation* by using some systematic scheme such as, for example, giving treatment A to those people with even birth dates, and treatment *B* to those with odd dates. Whilst in principle *unbiased*, problems arise because of the openness of the allocation system, and the consequent possibility of abuse.

Systematic error: A term most often used in a clinical laboratory to describe the difference in results caused by a *bias* of an assay. See also **intrinsic error**.

T

Tango's index: An index for summarizing the occurrences of cases of a disease in a stable geographical unit when these occurrences are grouped into discrete intervals. The index is given by

$$C = \mathbf{r}'\mathbf{A}\mathbf{r}$$

where $\mathbf{r}' = [r_1, \cdots, r_m]$ is the vector of relative frequencies of cases in successive periods, and $\mathbf{A}$ is an $m \times m$ matrix, the elements of which represent a measure of the closeness of intervals i and j. Can be used to detect *disease clusters* occuring over time. See also **scan statistic**.

Target population: The collection of individuals, items, measurements, etc., about which it is required to make inferences. Often the population actually sampled differs from the target population and this may result in misleading conclusions being made.

Taylor series expansion: The expression of a function, $f(x)$, as the sum of a polynomial and a remainder. Specifically given by

$$f(x) = f(a) + f'(a)(x-a) + f''(x-a)^2/2! + f'''(x-a)^3/3! + \cdots$$

where primes on f denote differentiation. Used in the *delta technique* for obtaining variances of functions of *random variables*.

Taylor's power law: A convenient method for finding an appropriate transformation of grouped data, to make them satisfy the homogeneity of variance assumption of techniques such as the *analysis of variance*. The method involves calculating the slope of the regression line of the logarithm of the group variances against the logarithm of the group means, i.e., b in the equation

$$\log_{10} s_i^2 = a + b \log_{10} \bar{x}_i$$

The value of $1 - b/2$ indicates the transformation needed, with non-zero values corresponding to a particular *power transformation*, and zero corresponding to a *logarithmic transformation*.

TD50: Abbreviation for **tumorigenic dose 50**.

Test statistic: A statistic used to assess a particular hypothesis in relation to some population. The essential requirement of such a statistic is a known distribution when the *null hypothesis* is true.

Tetrachoric correlation: An estimate of the correlation between two *random variables* having a *bivariate normal distribution*, obtained from the information from a double dichotomy of their bivariate distribution; that is, four counts giving the number of observations above and below a particular value for each variable. (See diagram.) Can be estimated by *maximum likelihood estimation*.

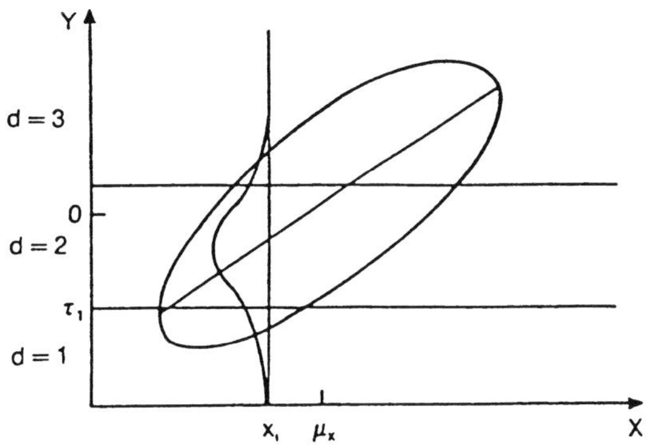

Fig 66 Tetrachoric correlation: an example of two ordered, categorical variables formed by imposing thresholds on underlying continuous variables.

Therapeutic trial: Synonym for **clinical trial**.

Three-group resistant line: A method of *linear regression* that is resistant to *outliers* and observations with large *influence*. Basically, the method involves dividing the data into three groups and finding the median of each group. A straight line is then fitted through these medians.

Three-period crossover design: A design in which two treatments, *A* and *B*, are given to subjects in the order *A*:*B*:*B* or *B*:*A*:*A*. Two sequence groups are formed by *random allocation*. The additional third observation period alleviates many of the problems associated with the analysis of the *two-period crossover design*. In particular, an appropriate three-period crossover design allows for use of all the data to estimate and test direct treatment effects even when *carryover effects* are present.

Threshold-crossing data: Measurements of the time when some variable of interest crosses a threshold value. Because patient examinations occur only periodically, the exact time of crossing the threshold is often unknown. In such cases it is only known that the time falls within a specified interval, so the observation is *interval censored.*

Threshold-crossing model: A model for a response that is a *binary variable*, z, which assumes that the value of the variable is determined by an observed *random variable*, **x**, and an unobservable random variable u, such that

$$\begin{aligned} z &= 1 \quad \text{if} \quad \mathbf{x}'\boldsymbol{\beta} + u \geq 0 \\ &= 0 \quad \text{otherwise} \end{aligned}$$

where $\boldsymbol{\beta}$ is a vector of parameters. In medical research z might be an observable binary indicator of health status, and $\mathbf{x}'\boldsymbol{\beta} + u$ a latent continuous variable determining health status.

Threshold limit value: The maximum permissible concentration of a chemical compound present in the air within a working area (as a gas, vapour or particulate matter) which, according to current knowledge, generally does not impair the health of the employee or cause undue annoyance.

Threshold model: A model that postulates that an effect occurs only above some threshold value. For example, a model that assumes that the effect of a drug is zero below some critical dose level.

Tied observations: A term usually applied to *ordinal variables* to indicate observations that take the same value on a variable.

Tietze–Potter method: A procedure for estimating the net discontinuation rates in studies of the effectiveness of contraceptives.

Time-dependent covariates: *Covariates* whose values change over time, as opposed to covariates whose values remain constant over time (*time independent covariates*). A pre-treatment measurement of some characteristic is an example of the latter, age and weight, examples of the former.

Time independent covariates: See **time-dependent covariates**.

Time series: Values of a variable recorded, usually at a regular interval, over a long period of time. The observed movement and fluctuations of many such series are composed of four different components, secular trend, seasonal variation, cyclical variation, and irregular variation. An example from medicine is the *incidence* of a disease recorded yearly over several decades. Such data usually require special methods for their analysis because of the presence of *serial correlation* between the separate observations. See also **autocorrelation, periodogram, harmonic analysis** and **spectral analysis**. (See Fig. 67 opposite.)

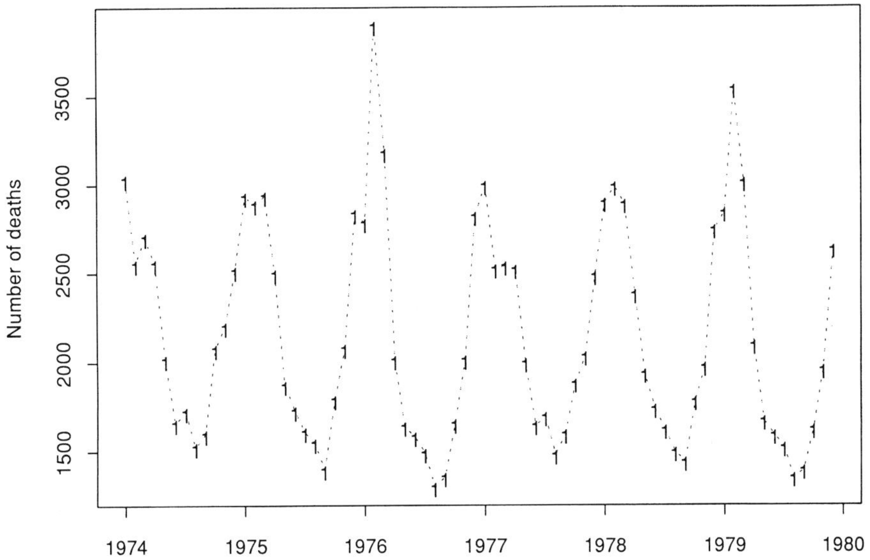

Fig 67 A time series of monthly deaths from lung cancer in the UK, 1974–1979.

Time tradeoff technique: See **Von Neumann–Morgensten standard gamble**.

Time varying covariates: Synonym for **time dependent covariates**.

Titration study: An investigation in which a patient receives a higher dose of a compound according to a set of predetermined rules, if he fails to achieve a satisfactory response at the current dose level and has not had any unacceptable reaction to the drug. Definition of a response is usually in terms of some objective physiological measurement, for example, the reduction of blood pressure below a certain level.

T_{max}: A measure traditionally used to compare treatments in *bioequivalence trials*. The measure is simply the time at which a patient's highest recorded value occurs. See also **C_{max}**.

Toeplitz matrix: A matrix in which the element in the *i*th row and *j*th column depends only on $|i - j|$. The *variance–covariance matrices* of *stationary series* have this property.

Tolerance: A term used in *stepwise regression* for the proportion of the sum of squares about the mean of an explanatory variable, not accounted for by other variables already included in the regression equation. Small values indicate possible *multicollinearity* problems.

Total matrix of sums of squares and cross products: See **multivariate analysis of variance**.

Total sum of squares: The sum of the squared deviations of all the observations from their mean.

Trace of a matrix: The sum of the elements on the main diagonal of a *square matrix*; usually denoted as tr(**A**). So, for example, if

$$\mathbf{A} = \begin{pmatrix} 3 & 2 \\ 4 & 1 \end{pmatrix} \text{then } \operatorname{tr}(\mathbf{A}) = 4.$$

Tracking: A term sometimes used in discussions of *longitudinal data*, to describe the ability to predict subsequent observations from earlier values. Informally, this implies that subjects that have, for example, the largest values of the response variable at the start of the study tend to continue to have the larger values. More formally, a population is said to track with respect to a particular observable characteristic if, for each individual, the *expected value* of the relevant deviation from the population mean remains unchanged over time.

Training set: See **discriminant analysis**.

Transformation: A change in the scale of measurement for some variable(s). Examples are the *square root transformation* and *logarithm transformation*.

Transition matrix: A matrix of probabilities, p_{ij}, representing either the probability of moving from state i to state j or the probability of state i conditional on state j. See also **Markov chain**.

Transition models: Models applied to *longitudinal data*, particularly when the response variable is a *binary variable*. In such models the response variable (or some function of it) is modelled in terms of a set of explanatory variables and of past responses. See also **population averaged models**.

Transmission probability: A term used primarily in investigations of the spread of AIDS for the probability of contracting infection from an HIV-infected partner in one intercourse.

Transmission rate: Synonym for **transmission probability**.

Trapezium rule: A simple rule for approximating the integral of a function, $f(x)$, between two limits, using the formula

$$\int_{a}^{a+h} f(x)\mathrm{d}x = \frac{1}{2}h[f(a) + f(a+h)]$$

See also **Gaussian quadrature**.

Trapezoidal rule: Synonym for **trapezium rule**.

Treatment allocation ratio: The ratio of the number of subjects allocated to the two treatments in a *clinical trial*. Equal allocation is most common in practice, but it may be advisable to allocate patients randomly in other ratios when comparing a new treatment with an old, or when one treatment is much more difficult or expensive to administer. The chance of detecting a real difference between the two treatments is not reduced much as long as the ratio is not more extreme than 2:1.

Treatment cross contamination: Any instance in which a patient assigned to receive a particular treatment in a *clinical trial* is exposed to one of the other treatments during the course of the trial.

Treatment–period interaction: Synonym for **carryover effect**.

Treatment received analysis: Analysing the results of a *clinical trial* by the treatment received by a patient rather then by the treatment allocated at randomization as in *intention-to-treat analysis*. Not to be recommended because patient *compliance* is very likely to be related to outcome.

Treatment trial: Synonym for **clinical trial**.

Tree: A term from a branch of mathematics known as *graph theory*, used to describe any set of straight-line segments joining pairs of points in some possibly multidimensional space, such that:

- every point is connected to every other point by a set of lines;
- each point is visited by at least one line;
- no closed circuits appear in the structure.

If the length of any segment is given by the distance between the two points it connects, the length of a tree is defined to be the sum of the lengths of its segments. Particularly important in some aspects of *multivariate analysis* is the *minimum spanning tree* of a set of n points, which is simply the tree of shortest length among all trees that could be constructed from these points. See also **dendrogram**.

Trend: Movement in one direction of the values of a variable over a period of time.

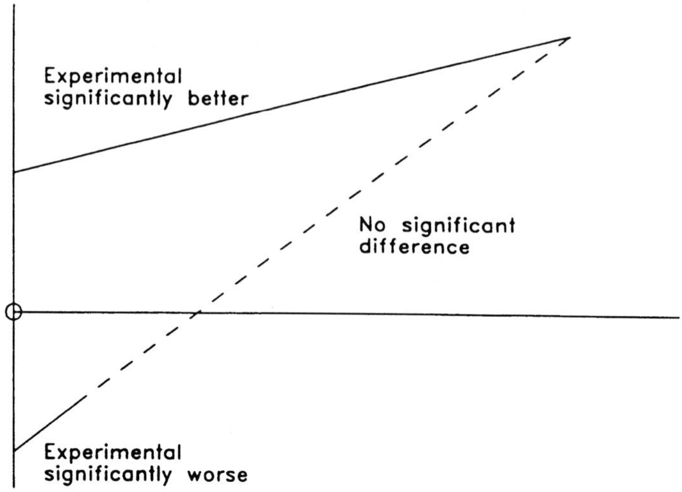

Fig 68 The triangular region of triangular test.

Triangular test: A term used for a particular type of *closed sequential design* in which the boundaries that control the procedure have the shape of a triangle, as shown in the diagram.

Trimmed mean: See **alpha-trimmed mean**.

Trohoc study: A term occasionally used for *retrospective study*, derived from spelling cohort backwards. To be avoided at all costs!

Truncated data: Data for which sample values larger (truncated on the right) or smaller (truncated on the left) than a fixed value are either not recorded or not observed. See also **censored observations**.

***t*-test**: See **Student's *t*-test**.

Tumorigenic dose 50 (TD50): The daily dose of a compound required to halve the probability of remaining tumourless at the end of a standardized lifetime.

Tumour lethality function: A term used in animal tumorigenicity experiments for the ratio of the death rates for tumour-bearing and tumour-free animals.

Turnbull estimator: A method for estimating the *survival function* for a set of *survival times* when the data contain *interval censored observations*. See also **product limit estimator**.

TWiST: A *quality-of-life* oriented endpoint for comparing therapies given by the *t*ime *wi*thout *s*ymptoms of disease and *t*oxicity of treatment. Calculated for each patient by subtracting from the overall time to symptomatic disease relapse, any previous time that the patient experiences treatment toxicity.

Two-armed bandit allocation: A procedure for forming treatment groups in a *clinical trial*, in which the probability of assigning a patient to a particular treatment is a function of the observed difference in outcomes of patients already enrolled in the trial. The motivation behind the procedure is to minimize the number of patients assigned to the inferior treatment. See also **minimization** and **play-the-winner rule**.

Two-by-two (2×2) contingency table: A *contingency table* with two rows and two columns formed from cross-classifying two *binary variables*. The general form of such a table is

		variable 1	
		0	1
variable 2	0	a	b
	1	c	d

Two-by-two(2×2) crossover design: See **crossover design**.

Two-dimensional contingency table: See **contingency table**.

Two-parameter exponential distribution: A *probability distribution* of the form

$$f(t) = \lambda e^{-\lambda(t-G)}, \quad t \geq G$$

The term G is known as the *guarantee time* and corresponds to the time during which no events can occur. In the analysis of *survival times*, for example, it would represent the minimum survival time.

Two-phase sampling: A sampling scheme involving two distinct phases, in the first of which information about particular variables of interest is collected on all members of the sample, and in the second, information about other variables is collected on a subsample of the individuals in the original sample. An example of where this type of sampling procedure might be useful is when estimating *prevalence* on the basis of results provided by a fallible, but inexpensive and easy to use, indicator of the true disease state of the sampled individuals. The diagnosis of a subsample of the individuals might then be validated through the use of an accurate diagnostic test. This type of sampling procedure is often wrongly referred to as *two-stage sampling*, which in fact involves a completely different design.

Two-sided test: A test where the *alternative hypothesis* is not directional, for example, that one population mean is not equal to another. See also **one-sided test**.

Two-stage sampling: A procedure most often used in the assessment of quality assurance before, during and after the manufacture of, for example, a drug product. Typically, this would involve randomly sampling a number of packages of some drug, and then sampling a number of tablets from each of these packages.

Two-stage stopping rule: A procedure sometimes used in *clinical trials* in which results are first examined after only a fraction of the planned number of subjects in each group have completed the trial. The relevant *test statistic* is calculated and the trial stopped if the difference between the treatments is significant at Stage-1 level α_1. Otherwise, additional subjects in each treatment group are recruited, the test statistic calculated once again and the groups compared at Stage-2 level α_2, where α_1 and α_2 are chosen to give an overall significance level of α.

Two-way classification: The classification of a set of observations according to two criteria, as, for example, in a *contingency table* constructed from two variables.

Type I error: The error that results when the *null hypothesis* is falsely rejected.

Type II error: The error that results when the *null hypothesis* is falsely accepted.

Type III error: It has been suggested by a number of authors that this term be used for identifying the poorer of two treatments as the better.

U

Unanimity rule: A requirement that all of a number of *diagnostic tests* yield positive results before declaring that a patient has a particular complaint. See also **majority rule**.

Unbalanced design: Synonym for **non-orthogonal design**.

Unbiased: See **bias**.

Uncertainty analysis: A method for assessing the variability in an outcome variable that is due to the uncertainty in estimating the values of the input parameters. A *sensitivity analysis* can extend an uncertainty analysis by identifying which input parameters are important in contributing to the prediction imprecision of the outcome variable. Consequently, a sensitivity analysis quantifies how changes in the values of the input parameters alter the value of the outcome variable.

Undirected graph: See **graph theory**.

Unidentified model: See **identification**.

Uniform distribution: The *probability distribution* of a *random variable* having constant probability over an interval. Specifically, the distribution function is given by

$$f(x) = \frac{1}{\beta - \alpha}, \quad \alpha < x < \beta$$

The mean of the distribution is $(\alpha + \beta)/2$ and the variance is $(\beta - \alpha)^2/12$. The most commonly encountered uniform distribution is one in which the parameters α and β take the values 0 and 1 respectively.

Uniformly most powerful test: A test of a given hypothesis that is at least as powerful as another for all values of the parameter under consideration, and more powerful for at least one value of the parameter.

Unimodal distribution: A *probability distribution* or *frequency distribution* having only a single mode.

Unit normal variable: Synonym for **standard normal variable**.

Univariate data: Data involving a single measurement on each subject or patient.

Universe: A little-used alternative term for **population**.

Unsupervised pattern recognition: See **pattern recognition**.

Unweighted means analysis: An approach to the analysis of two-way and higher-order *factorial designs* when there are an unequal number of observations in each cell. The analysis is based on cell means, using the *harmonic mean* of all cell frequencies as the sample size for all cells.

Up-and-down method: A method sometimes use for estimating the *lethal dose 50*. The method consists of the following steps: after a series of equally-spaced dosage levels is chosen, the first trial is performed at some dosage level and then trials take place sequentially. Each subsequent trial is performed at the next lower or the next higher dosage level according as the immediately preceeding trial did or did not evoke a positive response.

U-shaped distribution: A *probability distribution* or *frequency distribution* shaped more or less like a letter U, though not necessarily symmetrical. Such a

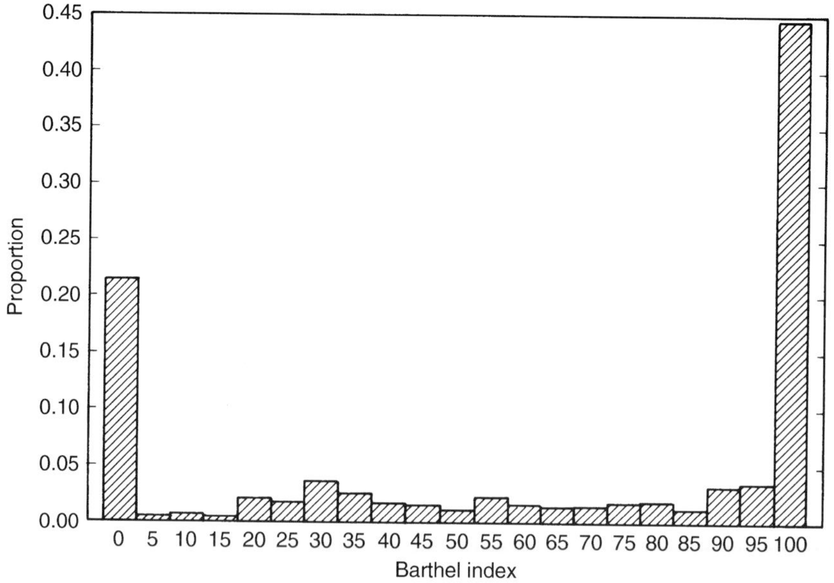

Fig 69 An example of a U-shaped distribution: distribution of the **Barthel index**.

distribution has its greatest frequencies at the two extremes of the range of the variable.

Utility analysis: A method for decision-making under uncertainty based on a set of axioms of rational behaviour.

V

Vague prior: A term used for the *prior distribution* in *Bayesian inference* in the situation when there is complete ignorance about the value of a parameter.

Validity: The extent to which a measuring instrument is measuring what was intended.

Validity checks: A part of *data editing* in which a check is made that only allowable values or codes are given for the answers to questions asked of subjects. A negative height, for example, would clearly not be an allowable value.

Variable: Some characteristic that differs from subject to subject or from time to time.

Variable selection: The problem of selecting subsets of variables, in *regression analysis*, that contain most of the relevant information in the full data set. See also **adequate subset, all subsets regression** and **selection methods in regression**.

Variance: In a population, the second *moment* about the mean. An *unbiased* estimator of the population value is provided by s^2, given by

$$s^2 = \frac{1}{n-1}\sum_{i=1}^{n}(x_i - \bar{x})^2$$

where $x_1, x_2, \cdots, x_n$ are the n sample observations and $\bar{x}$ is the sample mean.

Variance components: Variances of *random effect* terms in *linear models*. For example, in a simple *mixed model* for *longitudinal data*, both subject effects and error terms are random, and estimation of their variances is of some importance. In the case of a *balanced design*, estimation of these variances is usually achieved directly from the appropriate analysis of variance table by equating *mean squares* to their *expected values*. When the data are unbalanced, a variety of estimation methods might be used, although *maximum likelihood estimation* and *restricted maximum likelihood estimation* are most often used.

Variance–covariance matrix: A *symmetric matrix* in which the off-diagonal elements are the *covariances* (sample or population) of pairs of variables, and the elements on the main diagonal are the variances (sample or population) of the variables.

Variance inflation factor: An indicator of the effect the other explanatory variables have on the variance of a *regression coefficient* of a particular variable, given by the reciprocal of the square of the *multiple correlation coefficient* of the variable with the remaining variables.

Variance ratio distribution: Synonym for ***F*-distribution**.

Variance ratio test: Synonym for ***F*-test**.

Variance stabilizing transformations: Transformations designed to give approximate independence between mean and variance as a preliminary to, for example, *analysis of variance*. The *arc sine transformation* is an example.

Varimax rotation: A method for *factor rotation* that, by maximizing a particular function of the initial *factor loadings*, attempts to find a set of factors satisfying, approximately at least, *simple structure*.

Variogram: A graphical device used in the analysis of *time series*, *longitudinal studies*, and in particular in the analysis of *spatial data*. Consists of a plot of the variance of the difference in the observed variable values at separate times or sites against their distance apart. The plot is often helpful in describing the association among repeated values.

Vector: A matrix having only one row or column.

Venn diagram: A graphical representation of the extent to which two or more quantities or concepts are mutually inclusive and mutually exclusive.

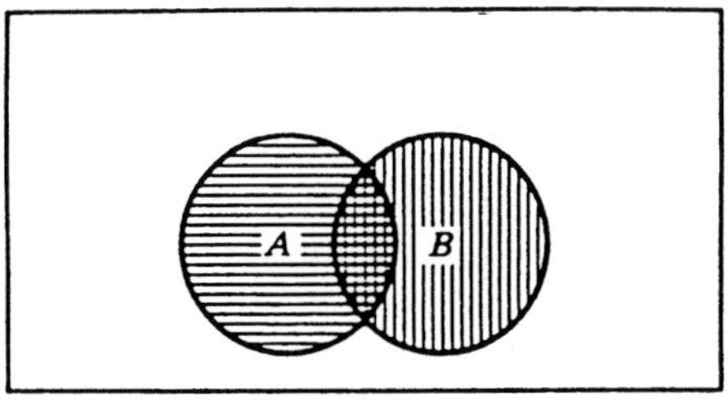

Fig 70 A Venn diagram: the intersection of the two sets A and B appears as the cross-hatched area

Virtually safe dose: The exposure level to some toxic agent corresponding to an acceptably small risk of suffering an ill-effect. From a regulatory perspective, this typically means an increased risk of no more than 10^{-6} or 10^{-4} above background.

Visual analogue scales: Scales used to measure quantities such as pain or satisfaction. The patient is shown a straight line, the ends of which are labelled with extreme states. They are then asked to mark the point on the line which represents their perception of their current state. For example, such a scale for pain might be

no pain –unbearable pain

See also **adjectival scales** and **semantic differential scale**.

Vital index: Synonym for **birth–death ratio**.

Vital statistics: A select group of statistical data concerned with events related to the life and death of human beings, for example, death rates and divorce rates.

Volunteer bias: A possible source of *bias* in *clinical trials* involving volunteers, but not involving *random allocation*, because of the known propensity of volunteers to respond better to treatment than other patients.

Von Bertalanffy's model: A general four-parameter model for response curves, given by

$$y = (\alpha^{(1-m)} - \theta e^{-\beta t})^{1/(1-m)}$$

By appropriate choice of values for the parameter m, a number of commonly used *growth curves* result. For example, when $m = 2$ it reduces to the *logistic growth model* with $\theta = -\gamma/\alpha$.

Von Neumann–Morgensten standard gamble: A suggested procedure for assessing the risk that seriously ill patients will take when offered treatment that offers potential benefit in *quality-of-life*, but with the tradeoff that there is a finite possibility that the patient may not survive the treatment. The patient is asked to consider the following situation:

> You have been suffering from angina for several years. As a result of your illness you experience severe chest pain after even minor physical exertion such as climbing the stairs, or walking one block in cold weather. You have been forced to quit your job and spend most days at home watching TV. Imagine that you are offered a possibility of an operation that will result in complete recovery from your illness. However the operation carries some risk. Specifically, there is a probability P that you will die during the

> course of the operation. How large must P be before you will decline the operation and choose to remain in your present state?

Because few patients are accustomed to dealing in probabilities, an alternative procedure called the *time tradeoff technique* is often suggested, which begins by estimating the likely remaining years of life for a healthy subject, using actuarial tables. The previous question is rephrased as follows:

> Imagine living the remainder of your natural span (an estimated number of years would be given) in your present state. Contrast this with the alternative that you remain in perfect health for fewer years. How many years would you sacrifice if you could have perfect health?

W

Wald's test: A test for the hypothesis that a vector of parameters, $\boldsymbol{\theta}' = [\theta_1, \theta_2, \cdots, \theta_m]$, is the *null vector*. The *test statistic* is

$$W = \hat{\boldsymbol{\theta}}' \mathbf{V}^{-1} \hat{\boldsymbol{\theta}}$$

where $\hat{\boldsymbol{\theta}}'$ contains the estimated parameter values and $\mathbf{V}$ is the asymptotic *variance–covariance matrix* of $\hat{\boldsymbol{\theta}}$. Under the hypothesis, W has an asymptotic *chi-squared distribution* with degrees of freedom equal to the number of parameters. See also **score test**.

Wald–Wolfowitz test: A *distribution-free method* for testing the *null hypothesis* that two samples come from identical populations. The test is based on a count of the number of *runs*.

Ward's method: A *agglomerative hierarchical clustering method* in which a sum-of-squares criterion is used to decide on which individuals or which clusters should be fused at each stage in the procedure. See also **single linkage, average linkage, complete linkage** and **K-means cluster analysis**.

Warning lines: Lines on a *control chart* indicating a mild degree of departure from a desired level of control.

Wash-out period: An interval introduced between the treatment periods in a *cross-over design* in an effort to eliminate possible *carryover effects*.

Weibull distribution: A *probability distribution* that occurs in the analysis of *survival data* and is given by

$$f(x) = \alpha\beta x^{\beta-1} e^{-\alpha x^{\beta}}, \quad x > 0$$

The parameters of the distribution, α and β, always have values greater than zero. An important feature of this distribution is that the corresponding *hazard function* can be made to increase with time, decrease with time, or remain constant, by a suitable choice of parameter values. In the special case where the failure rate is constant, i.e., $\beta = 1$, the Weibull distribution reduces to the *exponential distribution*.

Weighted average: An average of quantities to which have been attached a series of weights in order to make proper allowance for their relative importance. For example, a weighted arithmetic mean of a set of observations, $x_1, x_2, \cdots, x_n$, with weights, $w_1, w_2, \cdots, w_n$, is given by

$$\frac{\sum_{i=1}^{n} w_i x_i}{\sum_{i=1}^{n} w_i}$$

Weighted binomial distribution: A *probability distribution* of the form

$$f_{w(x)}(x) = \frac{w(x)B_n(x;p)}{\sum_{x=0}^{n} w(x)B_n(x;p)}$$

where $w(x) > 0\,(x = 1, 2, \cdots, n)$ is a positive weight function, and $B_n(x;p)$ is the *binomial distribution*. Such a distribution has been used in a variety of situations, including describing the distribution of the number of albino children in a family of size n.

Weighted kappa: A version of the *kappa coefficient* that permits disagreements between raters to be differentially weighted, to allow for differences in how serious such disagreements are judged to be.

Weighted least squares: A method of estimation in which estimates arise from minimizing a weighted sum of squares of the differences between the response variable and its predicted value in terms of the model of interest. Often used when the variance of the response variable is thought to change over the range of values of the explanatory variable(s), in which case the weights are generally taken as the reciprocals of the variance. See also **least squares** and **iteratively weighted least squares**.

Weight variation tests: Tests designed to ensure that manufacturers control the variation in the weight of the tablet form of drugs that they produce. The British Pharmacopoeia tests, for example, use a sample of 20 tablets from any batch. Each tablet is weighed singly and the average for 20 tablets found from the data. No tablet should deviate from the average by more than double the percentage given in the table, and not more than two tablets should deviate from the average by the tabulated percentage:

Average weight of tablet	**Percentage**
80 mg or less	10
between 80 mg and 250 mg	7.5
above 250 mg	5

Welch's statistic: A *test statistic* for use in testing the equality of a set of means in a *one-way design* where it cannot be assumed that the population variances are equal. The statistic is defined as

$$W = \frac{\sum_{i=1}^{g} w_i[(\bar{x}_i - \tilde{x})^2/(g-1)]}{1 + \frac{2(g-2)}{g^2-1}\sum_{i=1}^{g}[(1-w_i/u)^2(n_i-1)]}$$

where g is the number of groups, $\bar{x}_i$, $i = 1, 2, \cdots, g$ are the group means, $w_i = n_i/s_i^2$, with n_i being the number of observations in the ith group and s_i^2 being the variance of the ith group, $u = \sum_{i=1}^{g} w_i$ and $\tilde{x} = \sum_{i=1}^{g} w_i\bar{x}_i/u$. When all the population means are equal (even if the variances are unequal), W has, approximately, an *F-distribution* with $g - 1$ and f degrees of freedom, where f is defined by

$$\frac{1}{f} = \frac{3}{g^2 - 1}\sum_{i=1}^{g}[(1 - w_i/u)^2/(n_1 - 1)]$$

When there are only two groups, this approach reduces to the test discussed under the entry for *Behrens–Fisher problem.*

WE-test: A test of whether a set of *survival times*, $t_1, t_2, \cdots, t_n$, are from an *exponential distribution*. The *test statistic* is

$$WE = \frac{\sum_{i=1}^{n}(t_i - \bar{t})^2}{(\sum_{i=1}^{n} t_i)^2}$$

where $\bar{t}$ is the sample mean. *Critical values* of the test statistic have been tabulated.

White noise sequence: A sequence of independent *random variables* that all have a *normal distribution* with zero mean and the same variance.

Wilcoxon's rank sum test: An alternative name for the *Mann–Whitney test.*

Wilcoxon's signed rank test: A *distribution-free method* for testing the difference between two populations using matched samples. The test is based on the absolute differences of the pairs of observations in the two samples, ranked according to size, with each rank being given the sign of the original difference. The test statistic is the sum of the positive ranks.

Wilk's lambda: See **multivariate analysis of variance**.

Wilk's multivariate outlier test: A test for detecting *outliers* in *multivariate data* that assumes that the data arise from a *multivariate normal distribution*. The *test statistic* is

$$W_j = |\mathbf{A}^{(j)}|/|\mathbf{A}|$$

where

$$\mathbf{A} = \sum_{i=1}^{n}(\mathbf{x}_i - \bar{\mathbf{x}})(\mathbf{x}_i - \bar{\mathbf{x}})'$$

and $\mathbf{A}^{(j)}$ is the corresponding matrix with $\mathbf{x}_j$ removed from the sample. $\mathbf{x}_1, \cdots, \mathbf{x}_n$ are the n sample observations with *mean vector* $\bar{\mathbf{x}}$. The potential outlier is that point whose removal leads to the greatest reduction in $|\mathbf{A}|$. Tables of *critical values* are available.

William's agreement measure: An index of agreement that is useful for measuring the reliability of individual raters compared with a group. The index is the ratio of the proportion of agreement (across subjects) between the individual rater and the rest of the group to the average proportion of agreement between all pairs of raters in the rest of the group. Specifically, the index is calculated as

$$I_n = P_0/P_n$$

where

$$P_0 = \frac{1}{n}\sum_{j=1}^{n} P_{0,j}$$

and

$$P_n = \frac{2}{n(n-1)}\sum_{j<j'} P_{j,j'}$$

and $P_{j,j'}$ represents the proportion of observed agreements (over all subjects) between the raters j and j', with $j = 0$ indicating the individual rater of particular interest. The number of raters is n.

William's test: A test used for answering questions about the toxicity of substances and at what dose level any toxicity occurs. The test assumes that the mean response of the variate is a monotonic function of dose. To describe the details of the test, assume that k dose levels are to be compared with a control group and an upward trend in means is suspected. *Maximum likelihood estimation* is used to provide estimates of the means, $M_i, i = 1, \cdots, k$, for each dose group, which are found under the constraint $M_1 \leq M_2 \leq \cdots \leq M_k$ by

$$\hat{M}_i = \max_{1\leq u\leq i}\ \min_{i\leq v\leq k} \sum_{j=u}^{v} r_j X_j \Big/ \sum_{j=u}^{v} r_j$$

where X_i and r_i are the sample mean and sample size respectively for dose group i. The estimated within group variance, s^2, is obtained in the usual way from an *analysis of variance* of drug group. The *test statistic* is given by

$$t_k = (\hat{M}_k - X_0)(s^2/r_k + s^2/c)^{-\frac{1}{2}}$$

where X_0 and c are the control group sample mean and sample size. Critical values of t_k are available. The statistic t_k is tested first, and if it is significant, t_{k-1} is calculated in the same way and the process continued until a non-significant t_i is obtained for some dose i. The conclusion is then that there is a significant effect for dose levels $i + 1$ and above and no significant evidence of a dose effect for levels i and below.

Window width: See **kernel methods**.

Within groups matrix of sums of squares and cross products: See **multivariate analysis of variance**.

Within groups mean square: See **mean squares**.

Within groups sum of squares: See **analysis of variance**.

World Health Quarterly: See **sources of data**.

World Health Statistics Annual: See **sources of data**.

Wright's inbreeding coefficient: The probability that two allelic genes united in a zygote are both descended from a gene found in an ancestor common to both parents.

X

X^2-statistic: Most commonly used for the *test statistic* employed for assessing independence in a *contingency table*. For a two-dimensional table it is given by

$$X^2 = \sum \frac{(O - E)^2}{E}$$

where O represents an observed count and E an *expected frequency*.

Y

Yates' correction: When testing for independence in a *contingency table*, a continuous *probability distribution*, namely, the *chi-squared distribution*, is used as an approximation to the discrete probability of observed frequencies, namely, the *multinomial distribution*. To improve this approximation, Yates suggested a correction that involves subtracting 0.5 from the positive discrepancies (observed − expected) and adding 0.5 to the negative discrepancies before these values are squared in the calculation of the usual *chi-squared statistic*. If the sample size is large, the correction will have little effect on the value of the test statistic.

Youden's index: An index derived from the four counts, a, b, c, d, in a *two-by-two contingency table*, particularly one arising from the application of a *diagnostic test*. The index is given by

$$\frac{a}{a+c} + \frac{d}{b+d} - 1.$$

Essentially, the index seeks to combine information about the *sensitivity* and *specificity* of a test into a single number, a procedure not generally to be recommended.

Z

Zelen's single-consent design: An alternative to simple *random allocation* for forming treatment groups in a *clinical trial.* Begins with the set of N eligible patients. All N of these patients are then randomly subdivided into two groups, say G_1 and G_2, of sizes n_1 and n_2. The standard therapy is applied to all the patients assigned to G_1. The new therapy is assigned *only* to those patients in G_2 who consent to its use. The remaining patients who refuse the new treatment are treated with the standard therapy.

Z-scores: Synonym for **standard scores**.

z-test: A test for assessing hypotheses about population means when their variances are known. For example, for testing that the means of two populations having *normal distributions* are equal, i.e., $H_0 : \mu_1 = \mu_2$, when the variance of each population is known to be σ^2, the *test statistic* is

$$z = \frac{\bar{x}_1 - \bar{x}_2}{\sigma\sqrt{\frac{1}{n_1} + \frac{1}{n_2}}}$$

where $\bar{x}_1$ and $\bar{x}_2$ are the means of samples of size n_1 and n_2 from the two populations. If H_0 is true, z has a *standard normal distribution.* See also **Student's t-tests**.

***z* transformation**: See **Fisher's *z* transformation**.